CW01379234

Losing Weight with Atkins Diet Plan

A Beginner's Guide

Anna Adams

Table of Contents

Introduction: A Brief History of Diets 1

Low Carb Diets 6

What is the Atkins Diet? 9
    THE ATKINS APPROACH 10

The Science Behind Atkins - How it Works 20

Benefits of Atkins 22

Phases of the Atkins Diet 25
    PHASE 1 - INDUCTION 25
    PHASE 2 - ONGOING WEIGHT LOSS (OWL) 29
    PHASE 3 - PRE-MAINTENANCE 30
    PHASE 4 - LIFETIME MAINTENANCE 30

Eat This . . . Don't Eat That 32
    PHASE 1 - INDUCTION 32
    PHASE 2 - ONGOING WEIGHT LOSS 38
    PHASE 3 - PRE-MAINTENANCE 39
    PHASE 4 - LIFE MAINTENANCE 40

Avoid These Common Mistakes 41

Atkins 20 Meal Plans and Shopping Lists 46
    PHASE 1: INDUCTION 46

Phase Two - Ongoing Weight Loss 60

Phases 3 and 4 73

RECIPES FOR EACH PHASE 86
    PHASE 1 RECIPES 86
    PHASE 2 RECIPES 95
    PHASE 3 AND 4 RECIPES 100

A Final Word 105
About the Author 107

Introduction: A Brief History of Diets

Happy New Year!

Okay, maybe it's not actually January 1 (or maybe it is; there's one chance in 365, after all. And 366 in a leap year), but if you've decided that you're finally going to get serious and lose some weight, it's definitely going to be a new year for you.

Somewhere along the way, our world has turned into an environment of food. Temptation is everywhere: TV and radio ads boast of culinary delights of all kinds; books and magazines stimulate the appetite with delicious-sounding recipes--with pictures. Restaurants keep popping up in every city, and maybe worst of all, the fast food industry continues to thrive as we go about our busy lives. No wonder more than two-thirds of Americans are overweight!

So now we have a health crisis: just how are we going to get that weight off? And if we do manage to get it off, how will we be able to keep it off? Exercise could help. In fact, we should all be exercising regularly anyway, to keep our muscles toned and maintain our general health. But as far as losing weight, exercise by itself works slowly, if at all. No, the answer to the "how-do-I-lose-weight problem" lies in changing the way you eat. That's right, a diet. That's a four-letter word no one likes to hear.

Although you may think that the current obsession with weight is a modern preoccupation, the idea of dieting to lose weight goes far back into history. The first recorded dieter was King William I of England, or William the Conqueror. Apparently, this monarch was so overweight that it got to the point that he wasn't even able to mount a horse, much less ride one. Since this was definitely not very king-like, he decided to give up food and go on an all-liquid diet. His liquid of choice? Wine and spirits.

It's difficult to measure the success of his efforts to lose weight because the unfortunate king died in the same year that he began the diet. Ironically, his death was horse-related, so we know it must have worked to some degree.

In the 1800s, the poet Lord Byron may have been the first promoter of a celebrity diet. Apparently, he had something like a phobia about getting fat, and he ran through a series of weight loss campaigns. As a student, he limited himself to crackers and soda water with an occasional splurge on potatoes soaked in vinegar. Later he "advanced" to a breakfast of bread and green tea and a dinner of vegetables accompanied by a beverage of wine and seltzer water. To keep from getting hungry, he smoked cigars.

Lord Byron went on to adopt a diet of red cabbage and cider, and he apparently originated the idea of having a drink of water mixed with apple cider vinegar before meals. Sounds familiar, doesn't it? For the most part, Lord Byron was able to keep his weight under control with these crazy diets, but he paid a hefty price because he undermined his health and died at the age of 36.

And let's not forget the pudgy American President William Howard Taft, who, according to legend, got himself stuck in the White House bathtub and vowed that he would work on losing his excess weight. This story may or may not be true, but it is a fact that the 340-plus-pound president had special tubs made for him that would accommodate four full-grown men. So the idea of dieting is not a modern invention by any means.

One of the earliest diet books, published in 1810, was written by William Wadd, a surgeon whose concern was prompted by the death of a close friend. The autopsy showed an alarming amount of fat throughout his organs, including seven pounds around his heart.

The book Dr. Wadd wrote, *On Corpulence or Obesity Considered as a Disease*, was very helpful in its time and offered some sage advice on taking weight off. But there were also a few ideas that were just plain wacky. For example, Dr. Wadd admonished against drinking alcohol while overweight because he believed that the combination of alcohol and excessive fat could lead to spontaneous human combustion.

Following Dr. Wadd's book, in 1863, an undertaker named William Banting published a short pamphlet titled *Letter on Corpulence Addressed to the Public*. It became a huge success with new editions being popular even after Banting died. The premise of the book was very similar to the foundation of the Atkins diet: quality of food is more important than quantity for effectively losing weight. Banting's revolutionary diet proposed that quantity should be directed by a person's natural appetite, as long as the intake of food was high quality, healthfully speaking, and excluded starchy foods such as bread, cereals, etc.

Although the Banting diet had excellent results and was a great success among the public, members of the medical community criticized it because it was written by an outsider and went against the flow of scientific thinking at the time. Nevertheless, the diet continued to be followed by an appreciative public to the point that people in the UK who were trying to lose weight weren't dieting, but "banting." The word bant was even included in the Oxford dictionary until the early 1960s.

The years rolled on, and during the 1900s, a parade of diets came and went, and came again, and went again. Our great-grandmothers liked to say that they were "reducing." The diets included everything to calorie counting, fasting, eating certain "miracle foods," or any number of gimmicky trends.

Starting around the turn of the century, a man named Fletcher claimed that perfect health, perfect teeth, and ideal weight were all attainable if people would only chew their food more. This trend was called Fletcherism, and hundreds of people began chewing and chewing and chewing their food until it became liquid in their mouths. This practice may have resulted in some weight loss here and there, but it's more likely that any positive results were more from boredom and loss of appetite than the actual process of chewing.

The 1930s brought the Hay diet, where dieters were restricted from eating protein and starch in the same meal. The grapefruit diet also became popular during the 1930s, encouraging dieters to have half a grapefruit before every meal. In the 1950s, cabbage soup was introduced as another miracle food that would help in weight loss as long as that was all you ate at every meal. The grapefruit and cabbage soup diets both still resurface now and then even today.

In the early 1960s, a woman named Jean Nidetch invited a few friends into her home to support each other in their mutual efforts to lose weight. The number of friends continued to grow until it was too large to fit into her home, and soon the support-based Weight Watchers program was born.

Over time, many different weight loss trends have captured the public's attention. Some were serious, others plain wacky. The cotton ball diet actually caused the deaths of some of the people who tried it. (It seems that swallowing cotton balls to make yourself feel full can actually lead to a bowel obstruction.) There has been a peanut butter diet, an ice cream diet, a hot dog diet, a drinking man's diet, and a 7-day color diet. There have also been countless diet aids that include pills, appetite suppressing candy (Ayds), and diet "shakes" (Slimfast). And don't forget all the cleanses and detox programs that come and go.

But when all is said and done, the Atkins diet has given more people a successful outcome than most of the other diets and trends. Published in 1972, *Dr. Atkins' Diet Revolution* changed the way people thought about dieting. Instead of denying yourself so much food that you feel hungry and miserable, Dr. Atkins claimed that it was okay to eat as much of the right foods as you wanted until your appetite was satisfied. His famous motto is: "Eat right, not less." The only restriction on this diet is carbohydrates.

Dr. Atkins came to his conclusions after extensive research of studies that showed a link between lowered carb consumption and weight loss. He also noted that people who followed a carb-restricted diet did not experience any significant hunger. After the publication of his first book, Atkins published a few more, including *Dr. Atkins' New Diet Revolution, Dr. Atkins' New Carbohydrate Counter, Atkins for Life,* and some cookbooks.

There are two primary Atkins programs: Atkins 20 and Atkins 40. Atkins 20 is the original four-phase diet, and it is the go-to diet for people who have to lose 40 pounds or more. Atkins 40 is designed for people who have less than 40 pounds to lose, and it offers a bit more flexibility, such as eliminating the very strict Induction phase.

There are many other authors besides Dr. Atkins who have also written a variety of books that are designed to educate you about the Atkins program. This book is among that group, and it is ideal for beginners as it walks you through all the basics of the original Atkins 20 program, with a few upgrades that have developed since Dr. Atkins published his first book.

Not every diet is appropriate for every individual, and no diet book would be complete without advising you to check with your healthcare professional before starting on a diet plan. You don't want to risk your health; avoid this diet if you are under the age of eighteen, pregnant, or an extreme athlete.

Low Carb Diets

For decades, there has been a lot of controversy over the effectiveness and safety of low carb diets, especially those that promote high fat consumption to go along with the low carbs. The general consensus was that surely so much fat and cholesterol would lead to a higher risk of heart problems. And wouldn't such a high level of protein lead to the development of kidney stones? Why can't we just leave well enough alone and stick to the tried-and-true fat restricting, calorie-counting diets?

To address these concerns, scores of studies have been conducted over several decades, and results have shown that there is a substantial amount of evidence that the low-carb diets are not only safe and effective, but the traditional low-fat diet we mentioned earlier, while it has definitely been tried, it may be not as true as we once believed.

While the Atkins diet was one of the first to climb on board the low carbohydrate bandwagon, there have been many other diet plans developed that are based on lower consumption of carbohydrates. The Ketogenic diet is the most extreme, and some of the diets, including Atkins 20, base part of their programs on ketogenic principles. Then they tweak it a bit so that each diet takes a slightly different path toward weight loss. You may have heard of some of these diets: the Paleo (or Caveman) diet, South Beach diet, Dukan diet, and Sugar Busters.

To understand a low carb diet, it's only natural to begin with the carbohydrate itself. Carbohydrates are one of the essential nutrients within food that provide calories that we need for energy. Many of us may have forgotten our sixth grade science lesson where we learned that the starch components of carbohydrates turn into sugar. In fact, eating a simple potato can raise your blood sugar even more than eating plain sugar.

The carbohydrates that occur naturally in foods break down into simple sugars that convert to glucose during digestion. Your body uses glucose as fuel to function, but sometimes it can get out of control. As glucose levels in the bloodstream rise, the liver releases insulin to "escort" the glucose to the cells throughout the body. When there is extra glucose, it's either stored in the liver or muscles for a later time, or it's converted to fat. Controlling carbohydrates, especially refined carbs, has been shown to reduce the potential problems of out-of-control glucose, such as diabetes.

Carbohydrates are designated as simple or complex. Sugars are classified as simple carbohydrates. They earned this designation because they are made of only one or two molecules, which means that they move through the digestive system quickly and "simply."

Complex carbs, in contrast, move through the digestive process more slowly because they have multiple sugar molecules strung together in a chain, requiring a longer period of time to digest. Most complex carbohydrates are high in fiber, which requires even more time to digest, so they help you feel full for a longer period of time and keep your appetite from getting out of control. Foods that grow in the ground are the most common source of complex carbohydrates, and they also provide plenty of nutrients in addition to fiber, such as vitamins and minerals.

The principles that carbohydrate restricted diets are based on are built around the idea that lowering carbohydrate consumption decreases insulin levels, forcing the body to burn stored fat for energy. This burning of excess fat begins the process of weight loss. The low carb diets that are popular nowadays recommend a carbohydrate limit ranging from as low as 20 to 25 grams daily to 130 grams. Eating fewer than 30 grams means that the diet is considered ketogenic, also called a "very low carb" diet.

On the Atkins program, the type of carbohydrates is as important as the number. When deciding which carbohydrates are the "right" carbs, it's important to separate the simple carbs from the complex carbs. Another consideration to keep in mind is whether the carbohydrate is refined, like table sugar and white flour, or natural, like sugar in milk, fruits, and vegetables.

All low carb diets require you to stay away from refined carbohydrates, so you must avoid such favorites as white breads and crackers, white pasta, candy, cookies and other pastries, and sugary soft drinks. Those are obvious no-nos, but some manufactured products are sneaky and "hide" sugars and other carbs in their ingredients, so becoming a serious reader of nutrition labels must become part of your meal-planning regimen.

Generally speaking, most low carb diets are pretty similar in their focus: Eat protein, avoid carbohydrates. Some of these diets take you through graduated stages, beginning with a bare minimum of carbohydrates in the initial stage, then gradually adding more as your weight loss continues. The Atkins 20 approach recommends going through four phases in order to gradually change your whole way of eating.

What is the Atkins Diet?

Sometime in the early 1970s, cardiologist Robert C. Atkins, M.D. recognized that there seemed to be a connection between carbohydrates and weight gain with some people more prone than others to gaining weight because of carbohydrates. Rather than publish another ordinary diet book, he decided to set about creating a new way of eating that he felt would be an effective, quick way of losing weight.

Atkins understood that starving oneself to lose weight was inherently self-defeating, which was why many diets ended in failure. He conceived the principle "eat right, not less," and published his first book on the subject, *Dr. Atkins' Diet Revolution*, in 1972. It was met with mixed reviews, but a lot of people tried it and achieved remarkable results. The level of popularity remained at a simmer for a few years, then it built up to a full boil in the mid 1990s.

The Atkins diet recommends eating a certain number of carbs daily, starting out at a minimum level, which is basically a Ketogenic diet, then progressing through three more phases until you have retrained yourself on how you eat. In his book, Dr. Atkins proposed that a low carbohydrate lifestyle would re-calibrate the metabolism to burn more fat. The idea was to transition the body's metabolism to use fat rather than carbohydrates as its fuel of choice.

Although this idea met with a great deal of controversy in the medical field, subsequent studies on mice and humans have shown that reducing carbs in the diet does result in higher metabolic function. Of course, individual rates of success vary since genetics also play a role.

Since its introduction, controversy over the Atkins diet has continued, and some still exists today, despite many scientific studies and stories of success. For a long time, members of the medical community as a whole did not agree with or support Atkins claim that a diet consisting of low carbohydrates produces a "metabolic advantage," meaning that more calories are expended as our bodies burn fat simply because the fat-burning process itself actually requires more calories.

There were a number of studies to support this claim, including the ones with mice that definitely showed weight loss as a result of simply cutting down their intake of carbohydrates. But, according to Atkins' opponents, the so-called "metabolic advantage" was nothing but quackery. They cited other studies that argued against his claims, concluding that the lack of food choices created boredom in dieters and created a sense of tediousness. This supposedly impaired their appetite so that they weren't interested in eating so much, so of course they were losing weight.

Another problem the medical community had with the diet was the high volume of fat that is allowed in the diet, as opposed to the restricted fats of traditional diets. Most members of the health services community at first insisted that such a high volume of fat in the diet creates a higher risk for cardiovascular disease. But most studies of people on the Atkins diet have shown that their risks actually decreased.

The Atkins Approach

Under the Atkins plan, dieters keep track of the number of net carbs they are consuming, rather than the number of total carbs. The net carbs will generally amount to a lower number because grams of fiber are subtracted from the total carbs. This difference is because fiber does not have an impact on blood sugar, so it is not included in your count for carb consumption.

As an example, let's say you have half a cup of steamed broccoli. The carbohydrate counter you can find at Atkins-diet-advisor.com/carbohydrate-chart-html lists the carb count as 3.9 grams. If you find the grams of fiber it contains, you can subtract it from the total carbohydrates to get the net carbs. There are many online sources that list grams of fiber in foods. Even though the numbers tend to vary slightly, you can still get a reasonable idea of what to subtract to find your net carbs.

Finding the net carbs gets even easier when you're using a manufactured food product that is properly labeled (according to law) with all the nutrition facts. You won't even have to go to the Internet to find the carbohydrate and fiber counts because everything should be right there on the nutrition label. If the label indicates that the food contains sugar alcohols, you can subtract that number, too, from the total carbs.

The Atkins approach is founded on five principles:

Protein

While carbohydrates are limited, protein is an important part of every meal. It's essential for good health because it is necessary for growing and repairing tissue, producing hormones and enzymes to keep the body's engine running smoothly, and providing the necessary components for the body's organs, muscles, bones, skin, and hair, as well as the neurotransmitters in the brain.

Protein is the essential nutrient for building lean body mass. Moreover, people who don't have adequate protein in their diets experience lowered immunity; they are more prone to illness, and they take longer to recover. In addition, they may have problems with their skin, and injuries often take longer to heal.

Having sufficient protein in the diet also helps keep hunger under control. Protein is generally more satisfying, so with more protein and fewer carbohydrates in your daily diet, you feel fuller, so you are less likely to overeat. And eating protein actually assists in burning more calories, about double the amount that you burn from eating carbohydrates. Even a protein snack has been shown to have an effect on the appetite so that you don't feel the need to eat as much at the next meal.

Proteins are classified as either complete or incomplete. Complete proteins contain all the amino acids your body requires for good health, and they are available in animal products such as meat and dairy. Incomplete proteins have some of the necessary amino acids, but if you are not taking in any animal products, careful combining of incomplete proteins can provide all the amino acids you need.

Incomplete proteins come from plant products such as soy, brown rice, quinoa, nuts, seeds, and grains. Note that these foods also fall into the carbohydrate category. (That makes the Induction phase a little tricky for vegetarians_and virtually impossible for vegans. Not to worry, though; the Atkins plan is designed to be adaptable to personal requirements.)

Good fats

One reason that the Atkins approach has met with so much controversy is that it bucks the long-standing trend of limiting fat in the diet to lose weight. Ironically, during the same time period that people have tried to maintain low fat diets, the rate of obesity has been climbing higher and higher. Atkins theorized that the reason low fat diets haven't worked for everybody is that people were replacing fats with carbohydrates. This usually meant that they would eat more calories, because carbs just don't provide the same sense of satisfaction and fullness that fats do.

Manufactured "low fat" foods are not a solution to the problem, either. More often than not, a reduction in fat often means a reduction in flavor. So, to make up for that loss of flavor, other ingredients are usually added to a food when the fat is removed. A lot of the time the added ingredient is sugar. That's why many foods labeled as "low fat" can have just as many calories, sometimes even more, than the original version.

Fortunately, in recent years there has been a shift in how the public and many experts view fat in the diet, and the terms "good fats" and "bad fats" have been coined. Good fats are actually essential to a healthy diet. They protect organs, help the body stay warm, boost the body's insulin response, and act as an energy reserve. In addition, fat-soluble vitamins such as vitamin A, D, E, and K cannot be transported and absorbed by the body if there is not enough fat in the diet.

Besides all that, fat just feels good in your mouth and makes eating more enjoyable. Everyone knows how much more satisfying it is to add some butter to vegetables like broccoli and carrots, or maybe some bacon fat to plain green beans. Low-fat diets are often high-fail diets because without the enjoyability factor, it's just too hard to stick to. When you feel like you're being denied too many of the foods that make you happy, you're more likely to just give up and binge on everything you've been missing.

Unsaturated fats are classified as good fats, and they're broken down into monounsaturated fats and polyunsaturated fats. Many of your favorite foods and ingredients contain one or both of these types of fats, and, when eaten in moderate portions, they have been shown to help lower triglycerides and bad cholesterol (LDL) and raise good cholesterol (HDL) in the bloodstream, reducing risk of heart disease.

Monounsaturated fats are present in nuts and nut butters, avocados, olives, and oils such as canola, high oleic sunflower and safflower, sesame, olive, and peanut. Sources of polyunsaturated fats include other oils, such as corn oil, flaxseed, oil, and low oleic sunflower and safflower oils. Polyunsaturated fats are also found in walnuts, mayonnaise and some salad dressings, soft margarine, and fatty fish--especially salmon. Meats also contain a small degree of polyunsaturated fats, but saturated fats are the primary fat in meat.

Polyunsaturated fats are necessary for a number of bodily functions. They play a role in brain development and building nerve coverings and the membranes around cells. These functions are essential for normal growth and development. Polyunsaturated fats are also important in regulating metabolism, benefiting the reproductive system, clotting the blood, and supporting movement of muscles.

Polyunsaturated fats are broken up even further into omega-3 fatty acids and omega-6 fatty acids. These are designated as "essential" fatty acids because they are necessary in body functions, but they are not produced by the body. Both types of fatty acids have health benefits, but the omega-3 fatty acids have the most benefits for cardiovascular health. They help to lower triglycerides in the blood and reduce plaque buildup on the walls of the arteries, which are significant factors in developing a risk of heart attack. They are also important in helping to lower inflammation in the body.

Omega-3 fatty acids can be found in a limited number of food sources that include black walnuts, canola oil and un-hydrogenated soybean oil, flax seeds, chia seeds, and seafood, especially fatty cold water fish such as salmon.

Omega-6 fatty acids are also essential to a healthy diet, but our modern diets tend to include more omega-6 fatty acids than we need for optimum health. They're overly abundant because they're found in fast foods, many vegetable oils, mayonnaise, baked goods, processed foods, meats, dairy, eggs, and nuts and seeds. Although they do contribute health benefits, some omega-6 fatty acids have a tendency to trigger your body's inflammatory response, thereby counteracting the omega-3's efforts to reduce inflammation.

For that reason, it's important to make an effort to increase the amount of foods containing omega-3 while simultaneously decreasing, but not excluding, the amount of foods with omega-6. By substituting olive oil for corn and other vegetable oils, you're already on the way to creating a healthier balance. You should also avoid processed foods, which generally contain high levels of omega-6, and try to eat fatty fish twice a week.

The other type of fat, saturated fat, has been on the bad fat list in the past, but proponents of the Atkins diet maintain that even saturated fats have a place in a well-rounded diet. In some circles, they are coming into their own as a good fat. Saturated fats are found in animal products as well as some oils such as palm oil and coconut oil. It's easy to identify a saturated fat because it will become solid at room temperature and melt when heated.

The Atkins diet has included saturated fats since the early days, so there has always been a lot of criticism from many because saturated fat was believed to be a contributing factor in heart disease. Recently, however, researchers have revisited 72 published studies and conducted a new analysis on the data. The results showed that saturated fat actually had no effect on the heart. Moreover, saturated fats are necessary in building and protecting cells and supporting the immune system and liver function.

Although this is very encouraging, it's important to understand that the health benefits are directly proportionate to the *sensible* consumption of any type of fat. The Atkins diet recommendation for calories from saturated fat is not to exceed 20 percent of total daily calories. This contradicts statements from some Atkins dieters who have been known to brag that they could eat as much butter, bacon, cheese, and sour cream as they liked. Overindulgence will undoubtedly lead to health problems. And remember that all types of fat have nine calories per gram, so too much fat in the diet, even the Atkins diet, will ultimately sabotage your weight loss goals.

While most of the news about fats so far has been good news, there is a category of fats that is bad news. Transfats are bad news for your body and bad news for your health. Although a small percentage of natural transfats can be found in meat and dairy products, for the most part, transfats in our diets are not natural fats but unnatural fats manufactured by food chemists.

Transfats are most often found in hydrogenated or partially hydrogenated oils. The process of hydrogenating involves heating a natural fat to a very high temperature and then adding hydrogen. The reason they have become so widespread is their relatively low cost to produce, the fact that they help keep manufactured baked goods from crumbling, and their ability to last longer without spoiling.

Transfats are also present in most margarines and shortenings. Recently, some food manufacturers have recognized the public's negative response to the problem with transfats, and some of these products can now be found without transfats. You can find out whether a product is transfat-free by reading the label. If a product contains transfats, it must be listed on the label. It's the law.

Why are transfats so bad for you? Even small amounts raise triglycerides and LDL cholesterol, and they lower HDL cholesterol. These are the factors that are linked to a higher risk for heart disease and fatal heart attack. Recent studies have attempted to discover just how much transfat is safe to eat, and the conclusion was zero. Zip. Nada. In other words, even though it's difficult to completely avoid all the transfats out there, you should do your best to find healthy alternatives when they're available.

Low sugar

The third principle of the Atkins diet is following a low sugar lifestyle. As explained earlier, sugar is a carbohydrate, and refined sugar is nothing but empty calories. So followers of the Atkins plan must avoid eating anything with refined sugar or any of a number of sugar code names; sugar often tries to hide on an ingredient label under names like sucrose, glucose, galactose, dextrose, maltose, turbinado, cane juice, high fructose corn syrup (an especially evil offender), dextrose, fruit juice concentrate, honey, molasses… the list of sugars-in-disguise goes on and on. These sneaky added sugars show up in all kinds of processed foods from salad dressings, to sauces, to processed meats, to "low-fat" foods. Be aware.

For many people, cutting out sugar is a huge step in itself, and that step alone can lead to a significant weight loss. On average, Americans put away as much as 154 pounds of sugar per year in some form. In calories per day, that means that they are taking in 750 empty calories of sugar daily! As you know by now, this amount of sugar affects your insulin levels and inhibits fat-burning. In fact, the more sugar you eat, the more fat your body stores. By completely removing added sugars from your daily food plan, along with limiting the amount of natural sugars in fruits, vegetables, and other whole foods, you've made a giant leap toward managing your weight and achieving good health.

High fiber

The fourth principle of Atkins is including plenty of fiber in your diet. Fiber in foods is what gives you a sense of fullness, and in general, foods containing fiber are usually full of vitamins, minerals, and antioxidants. Although fiber is technically categorized as a carbohydrate, it doesn't fall under the to-be-avoided type of carbs because it isn't converted to glucose in the blood stream. Moreover, since fiber takes a longer time going through the digestive process, it actually slows down the rate of glucose moving into the bloodstream, so you are less likely to experience hunger or cravings.

There are many other benefits to having sufficient fiber in the diet. It does most of its work in the intestine as it adds bulk to the stool and smooths out the elimination process. It also helps to remove cholesterol, toxins, bile, and harmful bacteria in the intestine while feeding beneficial bacteria. All of these benefits support the immune system and help reduce inflammation.

Fiber is classified as either soluble or insoluble. Soluble fiber absorbs water from foods during the digestive process and is converted to a gel-like substance that slows down digestion. This improves the body's ability to control blood glucose, and it also lowers cholesterol. The type of soluble fiber you can eat depends on which phase of Atkins you are following. Soluble fiber is present in such foods as peas, lentils, beans, nuts, barley, oat bran, and some fruits and vegetables. Psyllium, a seed husk commonly used in fiber supplements, is also a good source of soluble fiber found in whole grains, bran, vegetables, and fiber supplements.

Insoluble fiber is undigestible, and it can be found in whole grains, bran, and many vegetables. Eating foods with a high fiber content will help to keep you "going" (aka, regular) by adding bulk to your stools. The bulk assists food in moving through the stomach and intestines at a faster rate. You can boost your intake of fiber in vegetables, salads, smoothies, etc. by adding insoluble fiber sources such as psyllium husks, bran, nuts, and seeds.

If eating more fiber is going to make a significant difference in your eating habits, start gradually and build up slowly so that your intestinal tract can adapt to the change. Otherwise, you may experience some bloating, cramps, and gas. In addition, be sure that you are getting plenty of water in your diet to help move the fiber so it can do its job.

Supplements

The final principle of the Atkins approach is to supplement your diet with vitamins and minerals. Dr. Atkins recognized that a diet of any type can mean that you are not getting all the nutrients you need from the food you eat. To ensure a good balance of nutrition, especially in the Induction phase, where fruit and grains are not allowed, he emphasized the importance of taking a good multivitamin with minerals. By supplementing your diet with the additional nutrients, you can avoid some of the problems that often occur with dieting, such as cravings, fatigue, and falling off the diet wagon.

The Science Behind Atkins--How it Works

So what kind of science is there to back up this whole idea of "metabolic advantage?" First of all, it's founded on a platform of body metabolism and fundamental biochemistry. Our bodies depend on fuel for energy and metabolic function, and that fuel comes from calories found in two nutrition sources: carbohydrates and fat. Unfortunately, our stored fat isn't called on for fuel nearly enough because we eat enough carbohydrates to not only supply plenty of fuel but also to store up fuel for the future in the form of fat.

Few would argue with the idea that over the past couple of generations our modern diet has deteriorated into a smorgasbord of too much refined sugar, white flour, processed foods, and other carbohydrate-dense garbage. Since the glucose provided by all those carbs is so plentiful, our bodies just burn that glucose to fuel our metabolic processes. The liver releases insulin, the hormone that converts any glucose that isn't needed into glycogen, which is then stored in the liver and muscles until it's needed again.

The glycogen stored in the liver can be returned to the blood as needed to give the metabolism an energy boost between meals and help keep blood sugar at a normal level. The muscles, on the other hand, do not share any of the glycogen they are storing, holding on to the glycogen until it's needed to help the muscles through high stress activities like workouts, sports, and other intense exercise.

But sometimes your metabolism doesn't require all the glucose and stored glycogen in your body. In that case, insulin will kick in to try to keep your blood sugar level under control, and the glucose from any carbohydrates that you eat will be turned into triglycerides and stored as fat. Unfortunately, while insulin does a good job of keeping blood sugar under control, it does have its limits, and sometimes your liver can't produce enough insulin to control an excess amount of glucose in the blood.

Too much insulin in the blood also keeps the body from burning stored fat because it senses that there is enough sugar to burn for energy. As a result, instead of burning fat, your body continues to add to your fat store, which Atkins terms the "insulin response." This is what is behind his claim that we must cut down on the amount of carbohydrates in our diets if we want to lose weight. When we take away most of the carbs, we still need fuel to function, so our body looks around for another source of calories to burn and, lo and behold, there's an abundant source of fuel being stored throughout the body as fat!

Now your surplus supplies of fat have a purpose other than padding your hips--energy! As you continue to burn the fat calories, the stores of fat become reduced, and so does your waistline. At the same time, you will lower your risk for developing heart disease and diabetes because, on a low-carbohydrate diet, your liver will not release as much insulin. You should also experience fewer cravings and less hunger.

There have been many published scientific studies that support these ideas. The studies use randomized controlled procedures that have involved both genders of varying ages, sizes, ethnicities, and health conditions. The studies have been published in highly regarded journals and other publications.

In spite of the high success factor of the Atkins diet, it's important to remember that there is no one-size-fits-all solution to losing weight. If you find that you are not losing weight, or you're losing weight too fast to be healthy, or you just feel terrible, Atkins may not be a good fit for you.

Benefits of Atkins

The all-encompassing benefit of the Atkins diet is what is known as "The Atkins Effect." It all boils down to how your body responds to switching from a sugar-burning to a fat-burning metabolism. Admittedly, not everyone will have the same response to the Atkins diet, or any diet for that matter, but if you have the type of metabolism that responds positively to the change, you'll be reaping all kinds of benefits:

You'll lose weight fast.

The Atkins approach is a double-whammy of weight loss because you're not only burning stored fat instead of glucose from carbohydrates, but you have less fat to be stored from excess glucose.

You'll be better able to keep the weight off.

Once you have reached your goal weight, you will have become very familiar with exactly how many carbohydrates your body can handle without losing or gaining weight. By staying close to this mark consistently, you will stay at your ideal weight for the rest of your life.

You'll experience less hunger.

The fats, proteins, and fiber of the Atkins diet all contribute to making you feel more satisfied between meals and less likely to head for the nearest snack. In addition, the absence of appetite-stimulating carbohydrates in your diet will play a part in keeping your hunger under control.

You'll reduce your insulin levels.

In addition, studies have shown an improvement in insulin sensitivity on a low carb diet, as opposed to the sensitivity becoming worse on a low fat diet.

You'll keep triglycerides at a safe level.

A healthy body needs some triglycerides, but a level that is too high can lead to an increased risk of heart disease. As long as your triglyceride level isn't a genetic problem, the Atkins diet will keep triglycerides under control.

You'll reduce fasting blood glucose levels.

As you know, too much glucose in the blood often leads to diabetes and other serious health problems. As long as the glucose numbers are normal, your risk for developing these problems will be much lower

You'll see improvement in your blood pressure.

In fact, a research study conducted at Duke University revealed that a group of subjects on the Atkins diet were more successful at lowering their blood pressure than members of another group that were trying to lose weight with Orlistat, a weight loss medication. It's good to know that you can lose weight without the expense and side effects of medication. Any significant weight loss will lower your blood pressure, but on the Atkins diet you will also be eating foods that contain high amounts of magnesium and potassium, nutrients that are known to reduce blood pressure.

Diabetics will see a reduction in their hemoglobin A1c levels.

This is the blood marker that reflects how well diabetes is being managed. Many diabetics on the Atkins diet have been able to either reduce or permanently discontinue their medications.

Your HDL cholesterol level will increase.

That's the good cholesterol, so the higher the number, the better.

You'll enjoy better overall health.

The Atkins approach reduces the factors that contribute to diseases such as diabetes, metabolic syndrome, and heart disease. In addition, the diet fulfills most nutrition requirements, with supplements added to reinforce the nutrition from the foods so that you can enjoy a long, lean, healthy life.

As you can see from this list of benefits, following the Atkins plan is a lose-win situation: you lose weight, but you win a better life!

Phases of the Atkins Diet

As we explained earlier, the Atkins 20 diet consists of four phases that gradually increase the number of calories you consume per day. If you don't have a lot of weight to lose, or you are a vegan, you may want to pass over the Induction phase and begin with Phase 2. Or you may want to stay with the Induction phase for three weeks, four weeks, even longer, until your goal weight is comfortably within reach. This diet was designed to be modified to accommodate individual needs.

Phase 1--Induction

The Induction phase is intended to last for a minimum of two weeks, and you can stay on this phase until you have only fifteen pounds left to go in your weight loss goal. This is the most restrictive phase, but then again, this phase is where you really get a boost on your weight loss. Don't be surprised (or alarmed) if you lose as much as fifteen pounds during the first two weeks. Of course, that's extreme, and most people are more likely to lose five to seven pounds.

Because the diet tends to have a diuretic effect at first, some of the early pounds lost will be water, but the fat will start coming off very soon, and it will continue to drop off as you progress through the phases. In the meantime, be sure you're getting plenty of hydration during this phase--go for eight 8 ounce glasses of water, broth, coffee, tea, or other no-carb beverages, but try to limit the non-water beverages.

Don't skip any meals because that will make your blood sugar start to react. You can choose to eat breakfast, lunch, and dinner, with a couple of low-carb snacks in between, or you can have four or five small meals instead. When you're awake, try not to go for more than six hours without putting something into your stomach. Don't let yourself become so hungry that you are tempted to become a diet dropout. If you feel any hunger, go ahead and have a snack. A handful of nuts or some olives and cheese might be all you need to tide you over to the next meal.

As you dive into the Induction phase of the diet, your metabolic engine is off to a running start during the process of switching from carb-burning to fat-burning. You need to help this process along by providing a minimum number of carbs, because that is what your body is used to looking for to use as fuel. Restrict yourself to no more than about 20 grams of carbohydrates a day in this phase, getting the majority of your calories from protein and fat. So you'll be eating at least six ounces of meats, fish, poultry, and eggs at each meal to satisfy your protein needs, and this will continue through all four phases of the program.

In this phase, about 12 to 15 of your daily net carbs will be from vegetables, focusing on those vegetables with the lowest carb counts. This level of carbohydrate restriction sets off a metabolic process known as ketosis. This is a normal state where your body responds to a lack of available glucose to use as energy, so it shifts to producing alternative energy molecules called ketones, which are produced when fat is metabolized. If you're burning fat, you're producing ketones.

Although there may be some unpleasant side effects from ketosis, after the first week or so you should feel amazing. You'll have more energy, more physical and mental stamina, and you'll experience less hunger. You can also avoid many of the side effects--bad breath, headache, irritability, constipation, lethargy, heart palpitations, and leg cramps--by drinking plenty of water throughout the day, as well as a bit of bouillon to replace salts.

Avoid skipping any meals, and maintain a moderate level of activity.

Some people think that ketosis is dangerous, but they're confusing it with an abnormal body condition with a similar name: ketoacidosis. This condition is indeed very serious, but it is not caused by dieting. By carefully following the Atkins eating plan, you'll be creating ketones that will work for you rather than against you.

To give you an idea of how your carb intake should progress, the Atkins program offers a "Carbohydrate Ladder" so you can easily see which carbohydrates to add as you progress through the phases. Since the protein and fats consumption won't vary from one phase to the next, it's good to have the carbohydrate ladder to simplify your menu planning and shopping. Note that *only* the first and second rungs include the carbs that are permissible while in the Induction phase. As you pass through each phase, refer to the carb ladder to see what you can be adding. Avoid eating all your daily carbs at one meal, but divvy them up throughout the day.

ATKINS CARBOHYDRATE LADDER

INDUCTION--PHASE 1

First rung: salad vegetables, leafy greens, and other low-carb vegetables labeled as "Foundation Vegetables" on the Atkins plan (See full list in section on what you may and may not eat)

Second rung: high-fat, low-carb dairy foods such as cream (not milk), sour cream, and many hard cheeses

ONGOING WEIGHT LOSS (OWL)--PHASE 2

Third rung: most nuts and seeds, with the exception of chestnuts

Fourth rung: melon (except for watermelon), cherries, and most berries

Fifth rung: whole milk yogurt, and now you can add fresh cheeses such as farmer's, ricotta, goat cheese, feta, and cottage cheese

Sixth rung: Bbeans, lentils, and other legumes, with the exception of peas

Seventh rung: tomato and vegetable juices

PRE-MAINTENANCE--PHASE 3 and LIFETIME MAINTENANCE--PHASE 4

Eighth rung: whole fruits (no dried fruit or fruit juices)

Ninth rung: vegetables with higher carb count, such as carrots, peas, and parsnips

Tenth rung: whole grains

Remember that everyone is different, and one person's tolerance for carbs may be higher or lower than another person's. If you find that introducing a new rung from the carb ladder results in gaining weight again, you may want to hold off on that rung until you're pretty consistently keeping the weight moving downward. On the other hand, if you seem to be losing the weight pretty rapidly, you can opt to move on to some of the carbohydrates further up the ladder. Just watch to see how each change affects your weight loss, and adjust as needed.

When attempting to lose weight, many people have the urge to check the scale daily, or even several times daily. But the scale is not necessarily your friend when you are dieting. You may or may not see the numbers going down rapidly, but if you feel that your pants waistline doesn't feel quite as tight as it did last week, you'll know you're heading in the right direction.

Resist the urge to weigh yourself every day, as it can be frustrating to see the numbers stall, or worse yet, go up a pound or two due to hormonal influences or other things going on in your body. If you restrict yourself to stepping on the scale about once a week (okay, twice, if you really can't help yourself), you're more likely to be happy with the numbers you see just above your toes.

Phase 2--Ongoing Weight Loss (OWL)

When Atkins refers to OWL, it's talking about Phase 2 of the plan, the Ongoing Weight Loss phase. In this phase, you will be able to increase your carbohydrate intake, but you should proceed with caution. Add only five grams of carbs per week, or every two weeks, or at whatever rate you're comfortable.

Introduce only one new food at a time and add only five grams of net carbs per week to your daily total. The carbohydrate ladder will be your guide as you add nuts, berries, cottage cheese, and some other foods you may have been missing. Just remember to keep balancing your carb consumption with protein and healthy fats.

If you find that a particular food seems to create cravings or hunger, it's better to take that one off the permitted list until the next phase. If the food continues to cause problems for you, you may have to eliminate it from your life permanently.

As you continue to add appropriate foods and increase your carb consumption, you will energize your metabolism and your weight will continue to drop. You should still be getting at least 12 to 15 grams of your daily net carbs from the foundation vegetables on the first rung of the carbohydrate ladder.

Be persistent in weighing and measuring yourself every week. You need to be able to keep track of how your body is responding so that you can find your personal balance of carbohydrates. It could level out at just 30 net grams, or it could go as high as 80 or even higher. It all depends on your individual makeup: your gender, your hormones, your age, your activity level, and other factors that are unique to each individual.

In general, you will remain on Phase 2 until you are about 10 pounds away from your goal. If you don't mind taking a little bit longer to get there, you can move on to Phase 3 earlier.

Phase 3--Pre-maintenance

As you transition into Phase 3, your goal should be in sight-- only about ten pounds to go! Now you are free to add even more foods to your daily diet, as long as you observe the effects of each new food you add. Continue to add five grams of net carbs per week to your daily total. If you notice a pound trying to creep back up, pause and rewind a little bit until your carb balance is back where it belongs.

Phase 4--Lifetime Maintenance

Once you've reached Phase 4, you've found your personal carbohydrate balance, what Atkins likes to call the ACE™, or Atkins Carbohydrate Equilibrium. This will be the balance of net carbs that will keep your weight stable for the rest of your life.

Your carb number may have stalled at 45, or you may have been able to climb all the way to 100 grams of net carbs per day without putting weight back on. You may even be able to eat more than that if you're very active. In any case, you have your own carbohydrate target, so now it's time to maintain it. That's why this phase is called the Life Maintenance phase.

It's important that you don't go crazy and do foolish things just because you've accomplished your goal. This was a hard-fought battle, but the war against weight gain will continue throughout your life. If you slip back into your old habits, you won't be able to slip into your new, smaller-sized clothes for very long.

Eat This... Don't Eat That

One thing that makes Atkins so easy to follow is the fact that every phase has a clearly defined list of food you should eat, and foods you shouldn't. When everything is outlined for you so specifically, it makes it so much easier to plan meals and shop for groceries. When you have a targeted goal of what to eat and what not to eat every day, it's harder to get distracted by all the tempting food displays when you shop. Use these lists to guide you in your food selections, and you're sure to stay on track.

PHASE 1--Induction

PROTEINS

This category will remain consistent through all four phases of the plan. Many people have the misconception that they're supposed to eat a large amount of protein on Atkins, but this is not true. The goal is to eat just enough protein to help you feel satisfied and stabilize your blood sugar so that, even though you're cutting out a considerable amount of carbs, you generally won't feel like you're being denied.

For the most part, you can eat as much as you like of all *meats*, *poultry, fish, and shellfish*. Now, don't be like some of those other people and take "eat as much as you like" as an invitation to gorge on protein. The protein is just part of your diet, and if you're getting enough fats and approved carbs, you should be quite satisfied with about four to six ounces of protein at a meal. (If you happen to be a big, burly man, you may need to take it up to eight ounces, but most people do fine with the smaller amount.)

Even though you are encouraged to eat enough protein to keep you satisfied, there are a few restrictions. Bacon and ham are allowed on Atkins, but they must not be the sugar-cured or honey-baked variety. If you're a fan of cold cuts, look for cured meats that have no added nitrates.

Most *seafood* is Atkins-friendly, but oysters and mussels have a higher count of carbohydrates, so they should be limited. Otherwise, enjoy the great variety of fish and shellfish, fresh or frozen.

Eggs are an excellent source of protein, so count on them as your breakfast protein on most days. You can eat them any style; try an omelette or frittata with some fresh spinach and mushrooms.

Some *cheese* is allowed on the Atkins 20 Induction phase. Cheese is an excellent source of protein and calcium, and it also contains some fat. But there are some carbs in cheese, so limit yourself to about three to four ounces of hard, aged cheese a day. One ounce is about the size of a one-inch cube, so three or four of those should be plenty. For cream cheese and blue cheeses, one ounce is about two tablespoons, and an ounce of grated parmesan cheese is about one tablespoon.

FATS AND OILS

Unlike the old school diets that restricted fats, you're expected to include fats in your weight loss plan on Atkins 20. Feel free to have butter on your vegetables, bacon drippings on your salad, and mayonnaise (check the label for added sugars) on your artichoke or fish. You can also use olive oil, preferably virgin or extra virgin, for dressing salads and vegetables, and you can sauté your foods in it. Some other vegetable oils are also permitted, including canola, grape seed, safflower, soybean, and sunflower. Walnut and sesame oils are good as dressings, but don't use them to cook with.

The healthiest oils to use are labeled "expeller pressed" or "cold pressed," which don't use toxins in processing the oils. When you cook with oils, make sure to watch that the temperature doesn't get too high, and you reach the smoke point. If you do, the oil will break down and form unhealthy chemicals. Not only that, the food you're cooking will probably taste pretty terrible.

FOUNDATION VEGETABLES

This section is the nuts and bolts of the Atkins plan, as this is where you'll be getting most of your carbs. Since 12 to 15 grams of net carbs per day should come from vegetables, the net carb count per serving of each vegetable should make it easy for you to plan your day's carb count.

½ cup raw alfalfa sprouts	0 net carbs
¼ medium steamed or boiled artichoke	4 net carbs
1 marinated artichoke	1 net carb
½ cup raw arugula	0.2 net carbs
6 spears cooked asparagus	1.9 net carbs
½ avocado	1.3 net carbs
½ cup cooked green beans	2.9 net carbs
½ cup cooked beet greens	1.8 net carbs ½ cup
chopped raw bell pepper, green	2.2 net carbs
½ cup chopped raw bell pepper, red	3 net carbs
½ cup cooked bok choy	0.4 net carbs
½ cup cooked broccoli	1.8 net carbs
3 stalks cooked broccolini	1.9 net carbs
½ cup cooked broccoli rabe	1.2 net carbs

½ cup cooked brussels sprouts	3.5 net carbs
½ cup cooked cabbage	2.7 net carbs
½ cup cooked cauliflower	1.7 net carbs
1 stalk raw celery	1 net carb
½ cup raw chicory greens	1 net carbs
½ cup cooked collard greens	1 net carb
½ cup sliced cucumber	1.6 net carbs
½ cup grated raw daikon radish	1.4 net carbs
1 dill pickle	1 net carb
½ cup cooked eggplant	2.3 net carbs
½ cup raw endive	0.1 net carbs
½ cup raw escarole	0.1 net carbs
½ cup raw fennel	1.8 net carbs
2 tablespoons minced raw garlic	5.3 net carbs
1 heart of palm	0.7 net carbs
½ cup raw jicama	2.6 net carbs
½ cup cooked kale	2.4 net carbs
½ cup cooked kohlrabi	4.6 net carbs
2 tablespoons cooked leeks	3.4 net carbs
½ cup shredded lettuce	0.5 net carbs
½ cup cooked okra (unbreaded)	1.8 net carbs
5 black olives	0.7 net carbs
5 green olives	0.1 net carbs
2 tablespoons chopped raw onion	2.4 net carbs
½ cup raw button mushrooms	0.8 net carbs

1 cooked portobello mushroom	2.6 net carbs
½ cup cooked, mashed pumpkin	4.7 net carbs
½ cup raw radicchio	0.7 net carbs
1 raw radish	0.2 net carbs
½ cup raw rhubarb	1.8 net carbs
½ cup drained sauerkraut	1.2 net carbs
½ cup chopped raw scallion	2.4 net carbs
2 tablespoons chopped raw shallots	3.4 net carbs
½ cup cooked snow peas	5.4 net carbs
½ cup cooked spinach	1 net carb
½ cup raw spinach	0.2 net carbs
½ cup cooked spaghetti squash	4 net carbs
½ cup yellow squash	2.6 net carbs
½ cup cooked Swiss chard	1.8 net carbs
1 small raw tomato	2.5 net carbs
10 raw cherry tomatoes	4.6 net carbs
½ cup cooked tomato	8.6 net carbs
½ cup cooked turnip	2.4 net carbs
½ cooked cup turnip greens	0.6 net carbs
½ cup raw watercress	0.1 net carbs
½ cup cooked zucchini	1.5 net carbs

You'll probably want to dress up your veggies and salads, so it's good to know that you're allowed to use prepared salad dressing with no more than two grams of net carbs per one to two tablespoons of dressing. Some of the dressings you can use: lemon or lime juice, red wine vinegar, balsamic vinegar, ranch, bleu cheese, Caesar, creamy Italian. Of course, the very best way to control the carbs is to make your own dressing. It's usually tastier, too.

WHAT CAN YOU DRINK?

As mentioned earlier, keeping hydrated is very important, and water, of course, is the best choice of beverage. You should drink at least eight cups of filtered water, spring water, mineral water, or tap water every day. But if you tend to get a little bored with plain water, and you want some variety, there are a number of other beverage choices you can make:

- Coffee *
- Tea--black, green, or herbal*
- Diet soda*
- Club soda
- Zero calorie flavored water and seltzer
- Heavy or light cream (up to three tablespoons per day)
- Soy or almond milk, unflavored

Clear bouillon or broth (check ingredients for added sugar)

*Watch your caffeine intake on coffee, tea, and soda. Try to limit yourself to one to two caffeinated beverages per day, then switch to decaf.

You can also use artificial sweeteners such as Splenda (sucralose), Sweet'N Low (saccharin), or stevia. These sweeteners do contain about one gram of net carbs, so be sure to take that into account. Diet sodas can also contain carbohydrates, so check your favorite drink to see if it's undermining your carb count.

ATKINS 20 INDUCTION PHASE NO-NOs

Since we've been talking about all the foods that you are allowed to eat, it's only right that we move on to what you should definitely not eat. (After all, it *is* a diet. A great diet, but a diet.)

When you're thinking protein, avoid any kind of imitation shellfish (think Krab) and meats processed with sugar, honey, or added nitrates and nitrites. The dairy products you should avoid in Phase 1 include cottage cheese, farmer's cheese and other fresh cheeses, and low fat or fat-free cheese.

There are several vegetables that have been left off the Acceptable Foods list for phase one because they're either starchy or they have a high sugar content. These include beets, carrots, corn, English peas, legumes, and winter squash (acorn, butternut, pumpkin).

Grains and grain products are also not permitted, so you need to avoid anything made with flour: bread, crackers, pastries, cereals, etc. Fruits and fruit juices are not allowed in Phase 1, and neither is alcohol. And it always bears repeating: NO ADDED SUGAR, and avoid transfats as much as possible (watch out, margarine).

PHASE 2--Ongoing Weight Loss

When you've reached the point you have about 15 pounds to lose, you can move on to Phase 2 and add a variety of new foods. From this point on, Atkins doesn't dictate the total number of net carbs you're allowed to have. Instead, you'll be adding acceptable foods in increments of five grams per week of net carbohydrates, as described earlier.

You'll be monitoring the effect that each addition will have on your weight loss, and if you stop losing weight, you'll need to go back to the previous level.

Dairy: Whole milk, ¾ cup heavy cream, 4 oz. plain yogurt, Greek or regular, 4 oz. ricotta cheese, 4 oz. cottage cheese, 5 oz. mozzarella cheese.

Seeds and nuts: 2 tablespoons hulled sunflower seeds, 3 tablespoons pumpkin seeds, 3 tablespoons sesame seeds, 2 tablespoons peanuts (not technically a nut, but a legume, but it seems to fit in this section), 2 tablespoons pecans, 2 tablespoons cashews, 2 tablespoons pistachios, 24 almonds, 10 macadamias, 6 Brazil nuts, 12 walnuts. Butters made from these nuts are also allowed.

Fruits: ¼ cup of any of these fresh berries: blackberry, boysenberry, blueberry, cranberry, gooseberry, raspberry, strawberry. You're also permitted ¼ cup of cubed honeydew melon or cantaloupe.

Juices: 2 tablespoons of lemon or lime juice, 4 oz. tomato or vegetable juice (such as V8).

Legumes: ¼ cup of the following: black beans, chick peas, Great Northern beans, kidney beans, lentils, lima beans, navy beans, pinto beans.

Other: coconut milk, almond milk (unsweetened), soy milk (unsweetened), shirataki noodles, specialty low carb foods such as Atkins bars and shakes.

PHASE 3--Pre-Maintenance

Now you can add fruits, whole grains, and sweetish or starchy vegetables that you've been missing:

Vegetables: ½ cup sliced beets, ½ cup corn, ½ cup acorn or butternut squash, ½ cup peas, 1 medium carrot, ½ cup cubed rutabaga, ½ cup sliced parsnip, ½ medium sweet potato, ½ small baked potato.

Fruits: 1 small banana, ½ cup fresh pineapple chunks, ½ cup shredded coconut, 1 medium pear, 1 fresh fig, 3 fresh dates, ¼ cup fresh cherries, 1 navel orange, ½ cup watermelon cubes, ½ cup red grapes, ¼ cup pomegranate arils (aka seeds), ½ cup cubed mango, ½ cup sliced papaya, 3 medium apricots, 1 medium plum, ½ medium grapefruit, ½ cup cubed guava, 1 kiwi, 1 small peach, 1 clementine, ½ apple.

Grains: ½ cup barley, ½ cup grits, ½ cup millet, 2 tablespoons oat bran, ½ cup oatmeal (steel cut), ½ cup rolled oatmeal, ¼ cup polenta, ¼ cup quinoa, ½ cup brown rice, 2 tablespoons wheat germ, 1 slice whole wheat bread, ½ cup whole wheat pasta.

Anything made with refined white flour is still on the list of unacceptable foods. In fact, you may just as well say goodbye to those foods forever. White flour is not your friend.

PHASE 4--Life Maintenance

After all the lists in this section, you'll be glad to know that you're eating on Phase 4 is just going to be a continuation of the three previous phases. Now you can eat whatever makes you happy, as long as you stay within the limits of your personal carb balance. Continue to avoid rich, high-sugar desserts, simple carbohydrates (added sugar, refined white flour), food containing transfats, or too much alcohol.

Avoid These Common Mistakes

Even when you have the best intentions, it's only human to make a mistake here and there, and that's just as true when you're following a plan to lose weight. To make it easier for you, we've made a list of some of the mistakes that others have made so that you have a better chance of avoiding them and saving yourself some frustrating stalls, or heaven forbid, backslides.

First mistake: Neglecting to keep a record of your progress.

Buy yourself one of those nifty notebook/journals that you see everywhere, and keep track of how much food you eat every day, along with your daily total of net carbs. You also need to keep a weekly record of your weight and measurements.

Second mistake: Under- or overestimating your protein requirements.

Every meal should include four to six ounces of protein. Eating more or less, or none at all, will lead to hunger, cravings, and unreliable weight loss.

Third mistake: Not eating your veggies.

Remember, 12 to 15 grams of your net carbs should be coming from the foundation vegetables. While you may think that that doesn't sound like much, in fact it's the equivalent of about six cups of the leafy salad greens plus two cups of the cooked vegetables. That's quite a hefty amount, but if you're dividing your vegetables between breakfast, lunch, and dinner, it's comfortably doable.

Losing Weight with Atkins Diet Plan: A Beginner's Guide

Fourth mistake: Keeping track of total carbs, rather than net carbs.

Remember, most fiber doesn't count because it doesn't raise your blood sugar. If you remember to subtract the grams of fiber from the total count, you'll be able to eat more. Another mistake is forgetting to count the carbs in condiments such as sugar substitutes, lemon juice, etc. If a food contains carbohydrates, they count. And don't think that just because a chocolate croissant is under the carb limit you can eat that and have no other carbs for the day. That's just asking for a boatload of trouble. On the other hand, don't buy into the idea that "if low carb is good, no carb is better." If you restrict yourself to eating only fat and protein, you'll be heading down the road to bad health. Atkins' website has all kinds of free tools to help you stay on track. Check out the Atkins Carb Counter to help you keep track of the net carbs you're eating.

Fifth mistake: Not getting your recommended amount of fluid.

Just about every health guru recommends eight cups of liquid, the greater part of which should be water, every day. If you're very active, or you're living in a warm environment, you need even more. You can supplement with coffee, tea, and other acceptable drinks, but you should keep them down to about two cups. Some people actually believe that less water means that they will weigh less when they step on the scale, but it's actually the opposite. When your body isn't getting the hydration it needs, it will start to retain fluids to protect from dehydration. So you'll actually see a bigger number when it's time to check your weight.

Sixth mistake: Weighing yourself too much or not enough.

As mentioned earlier, weighing yourself every day is unnecessary and often quite frustrating. Your weight can go up and down as much as five pounds during a day, so a daily scale hop is not a good reflection of how you're doing. Furthermore, if you are adopting a new exercise routine at the same time as you're dieting, you're probably adding muscle; if you weigh the same volume of muscle and fat, the muscle will be about ⅕ heavier. So it's best to take that into consideration, and take your measurements weekly to get the whole picture. If the inches are going down while the pounds aren't budging, you'll know it's muscle. It won't be long before your progress also shows up on the scale. That being said, it's still important that you do weigh yourself regularly, especially as you add carbs. If you see the numbers start to creep back up, you know the carb count is getting too high.

Seventh mistake: Cutting out salt.

Unless you're under doctor's orders, you shouldn't take salt out of your diet. The process of transitioning from a carb-burning to a fat-burning metabolism naturally has a diuretic effect, so you need the salt to avoid some of the initial side effects that occur as you lose electrolytes and minerals. Sprinkle a little table salt on your eggs, some soy sauce on your stir-fry, or have a little broth to avoid muscle cramps, lightheadedness, weakness, or headaches as you adjust. Just don't overdo it.

Eighth mistake: Being too careful with fat.

Since your goal is to burn body fat, you must have some fat in your diet to get the process going. As long as you're controlling your carbs, most of the fat you eat will become fuel. You need both protein and fat to help keep you feeling satisfied and curb your appetite. You also need the calories from fat to keep your metabolism from going into "starvation" mode and slowing down.

Ninth mistake: Not recognizing foods with hidden carbs.

It's surprising how many food products are out there that contain added sugars and carbs. Low calorie and low fat products are especially prone to add sugars to enhance taste. It's very important to read product labels (the ingredient section, not the nutrition facts) to find hidden carbs.

Tenth mistake: Choosing low carb products other than Atkins.

While some of these products might sound good and safe to eat, they haven't undergone the Atkins testing for blood sugar impact. Most of the Atkins products are acceptable for all phases, including induction.

Eleventh mistake: Thinking that the Induction phase is the entire program.

Although you can stay in Phase 1 for an extended period of time, it's important to move forward as you approach your weight loss goal. Your ultimate objective is to get to a point where you're eating the ideal balance of carbs, proteins, and fats so that you can maintain this diet for the rest of your life. It's unrealistic to think that anyone will be able to continue with 20 grams of net carbs indefinitely.

Twelfth mistake: Failing to continue to count the net carbs through all the phases.

Yes, it can get tiresome looking up to see how many carbs are in a certain food. But if you start to rely on memory, intuition, or your gut, you're more likely to have your carb consumption go beyond the range it needs to be in.

Thirteenth mistake: Not getting enough to eat.

Some people are so ecstatic at the speed of their weight loss on Atkins that they want to go even faster. They cut down even further on carbs, but also on protein and fats. This is a mistake because you're not getting enough calories to maintain your lean muscle mass.

A single mistake now and then is not going to erase all the progress you've made, but we should add a fourteenth mistake: giving up after one mistake. No one expects you to be a superman or superwoman, so don't expect it of yourself. If you have a little slip-up one day (and let's face it, who doesn't?) just take a deep breath and move forward again. Don't wait, because it only takes a couple of days for your body to begin burning those carbs for fuel again. The biggest mistake of all is giving up.

Atkins 20 Meal Plans and Shopping Lists

Although Atkins is designed to be customized for individual preferences, some people feel a little lost when it's time to plan their meals for the week and go shopping. The meal plans in this section are intended to be a guide as you eat and shop your way through the four phases. Each phase contains meal plans that are on the more conservative side of the carb limit, but you have the freedom to add foods and quantities as appropriate for you.

Once you have familiarized yourself with the basic framework of the meal plans offered here, you will have the know-how to do your own thing. The point is to make every meal and snack enjoyable. No one is meant to suffer on Atkins.

Phase 1: Induction

Week One

SUNDAY BREAKFAST:

2-egg omelette with spinach and cheddar cheese;
3 slices Canadian bacon;
1 cup coffee
5 net carbs

SUNDAY LUNCH

1 cup chicken broth;
1 six-ounce chicken breast, grilled;

1 cup heart of romaine salad with 1 tablespoon vinaigrette dressing; iced mineral water
4 net carbs

SUNDAY DINNER

1 cup mixed greens with blue cheese dressing;
1 ham steak (6 ounces);
½ cup green beans tossed with bacon drippings;
iced tea with lemon
6 net carbs

SNACKS

5 black olives with 1 wedge Laughing Cow cheese 2nc
3 ounces small shrimp with lemon juice 1nc

* * *

MONDAY BREAKFAST

2-egg Greek omelette with ½ cup spinach and 2 ounces feta cheese;
½ small tomato, sliced;
1 cup coffee 3.4 nc

MONDAY LUNCH

6 ounces baked turkey meatballs;
green beans drizzled with bacon drippings;
1 cup mixed greens with 2 teaspoons ranch dressing; diet soda
8.9 nc

MONDAY DINNER

6 ounces roast beef, au jus;
1/2 cup mashed cauliflower with butter; 1 cup mixed greens with vinaigrette dressing;
iced water   6 nc

SNACKS

1/2 small cucumber, sliced   2.5 nc
1 cup chicken broth   1 nc

***

TUESDAY BREAKFAST

2 eggs, scrambled;
1 link sausage,
1/2 cup sliced cherry tomatoes;
1 cup cinnamon tea   2 nc

TUESDAY LUNCH

Chef salad: 3 cups mixed greens with ham, turkey, chopped hard boiled egg, 1 ounce crumbled bleu cheese, and crumbled bacon (2 slices) with 2 teaspoons vinaigrette dressing;
diet soda   7.5 nc

TUESDAY DINNER

6 ounces tuna steak, grilled;

½ cup artichoke hearts packed in water, steamed; salad with 2 cups mixed greens with 2 teaspoons bleu cheese dressing; iced tea   6 nc

SNACKS

1 ounce cheddar cheese   1 nc
chorizo with lemon mayo dip (see recipe)   2.8 nc

**

WEDNESDAY BREAKFAST

Broccoli and cheese mini omelettes (see recipe);
green tea   2.5 nc

WEDNESDAY LUNCH

Cobb salad with 3 cups mixed greens, 4 ounces cooked chicken, 1 slice crumbled bacon, ½ cubed avocado, 1 ounce crumbled bleu cheese, and 2 teaspoons vinaigrette dressing;
iced mineral water   8 nc

WEDNESDAY DINNER

Creamy soup with turkey meatballs (see recipe);
1 cup mixed greens with vinaigrette dressing;
iced tea   4 nc

SNACKS
½ cup fennel and 1 tablespoon sour cream dip   3 nc

½ cup sugar-free gelatin; 2 tablespoons whipped heavy cream
                                               1.5 nc

***

THURSDAY BREAKFAST

2 scrambled eggs mixed with 3 ounces crumbled,
cooked turkey sausage;
½ small tomato, sliced;
coffee   3 nc

THURSDAY LUNCH

Shrimp fried "rice" (see recipe);
½ cup cooked broccoli;
iced water   9 nc

THURSDAY DINNER

1 six-ounce pork chop, grilled;
½ cup zucchini, sautéed or roasted;
2 cups mixed greens salad with 2 teaspoons vinaigrette dressing;
diet soda   7.7 nc

SNACKS

1 ounce Monterey Jack cheese   1 nc
1 deviled egg   0.5 nc

***

FRIDAY BREAKFAST

2 poached eggs over ½ cup sautéed spinach;
2 strips bacon;
coffee   2 nc

FRIDAY LUNCH

1 cup chicken, beef, or vegetable broth;
salad with 2 cups baby spinach leaves, 4 ounces chopped roast turkey, 1 slice bacon, crumbled, 2 teaspoons ranch dressing;
iced water with lemon wedge;
diet soda   4nc

FRIDAY DINNER

6 ounces broiled lamb chops;
1 cup roasted cauliflower;
1 cup mixed greens salad with 2 teaspoons bleu cheese dressing;
iced tea with lemon wedge   6 nc

SNACKS

1 ounce string cheese with 5 black olives   2 nc
½ avocado   2 nc

***

SATURDAY BREAKFAST

Mexican-style eggs on Canadian bacon 2.5;
½ cup sliced cherry tomatoes;
coffee   4.5 nc

SATURDAY LUNCH

6 oz. canned salmon mixed with 2 tablespoons mayo, 1 tablespoon chopped parsley, and ½ cup
chopped cucumber;
2 cups mixed greens with ¼ cup red chopped red bell pepper and
2 tablespoons vinaigrette   5.5 nc

SATURDAY DINNER

crispy carnitas (see recipe);
½ sliced avocado;
club soda   8.7 nc

SNACKS

1 deviled egg   0.5 nc
2 tablespoons cream cheese with celery sticks   2 nc

WEEK ONE SHOPPING LIST

MEATS/SEAFOOD: no-sugar bacon, chicken breast, ham steak, cooked small shrimp, ground turkey, beef roast, sausage links (not sugar cured), roast turkey, tuna steak, beef and pork chorizo, turkey sausage, medium shrimp, pork chop, lamb chops, Canadian bacon, 3-4 pound boneless pork shoulder

PRODUCE: spinach, hearts of romaine, mixed greens, green beans, lemon, spinach, tomatoes, cauliflower, cucumber, cherry tomatoes artichoke hearts packed in water, white mushrooms, fennel, sour cream, green onions, zucchini, red bell pepper, pear, hazelnuts

EGGS AND DAIRY: eggs, cheddar cheese, Laughing Cow cheese, feta cheese, Monterey Jack cheese, string cheese, heavy cream

OTHER: chicken broth, vinegar, olive oil, bleu cheese dressing, ranch dressing, black olives, mayonnaise, chicken bouillon powder, sugar free gelatin dessert, sesame oil, canned salmon, cumin, chili powder, bay leaves, garlic, cinnamon sticks, arugula

WEEK TWO

SUNDAY BREAKFAST:

Egg and sausage nibbles (see recipe);
¼ sliced cucumber;
coffee   6 nc

SUNDAY LUNCH

Shrimp salad with 2 cups mixed salad greens, 6 ounces chopped cooked shrimp, ½ cup chopped bell
pepper, chopped parsley, and 2 teaspoons vinaigrette dressing;
iced water   nc 7

SUNDAY DINNER

6 ounces grilled flat iron steak;
1 cup sautéed sliced zucchini and mushrooms;
salad with 1 cup arugula, ½ cup sliced cucumber, and 2 teaspoons ranch dressing;
iced tea with lemon   5 nc

SNACKS

1 ounce Swiss cheese   1 nc
celery sticks   1.5 nc

                              ***

MONDAY BREAKFAST

2 poached eggs on 2 slices Canadian bacon;
½ small tomato, sliced;
herbal tea   2 nc

MONDAY LUNCH

1 6-oz ground beef patty topped with 2 tablespoons bleu cheese
and ½ cup sliced cherry tomatoes;
2 cups mixed greens with vinaigrette dressing   7 nc

MONDAY DINNER

6 ounces halibut, pan-fried;
1 serving faux mashed potatoes (see recipe section); 1 cup mixed
greens salad with 2 tablespoons vinaigrette;
decaf coffee   9 nc

SNACKS

2 tablespoons cream cheese rolled in 2 ounces ham slices with 2
dill pickle spears   2.5 nc

                              ***

TUESDAY BREAKFAST

2 eggs, scrambled, topped with 1 ounce grated
Monterey Jack cheese, 1 tablespoon green salsa, and
1 tablespoon sour cream; 2 links of turkey sausage;
coffee   4 nc

TUESDAY LUNCH

6 ounces tuna salad in ½ avocado; 2 cups spinach
salad with 2 teaspoons vinaigrette dressing;
club soda   6 nc

TUESDAY DINNER

6 ounces roast pork tenderloin;
3 cups romaine salad with 2 tablespoons crumbled bleu cheese,
2 tablespoons sun-dried tomatoes packed in olive oil,
2 tablespoons lite balsamic vinaigrette;
iced tea   7 nc

SNACKS

5 black olives	1 nc
½ cup sliced cucumber with	1 oz.
Swiss cheese	1 nc

***

WEDNESDAY BREAKFAST

two poached eggs with one small tomato, sliced, and 2
tablespoons hollandaise sauce; 2 slices Canadian
bacon, yerba mate tea   4 nc

WEDNESDAY LUNCH

one cup chicken broth;
chef salad with ham, turkey, hard boiled egg, 1 ounce grated cheddar cheese, grated, over 3 cups mixed greens
2 teaspoons vinaigrette dressing   7.5 nc

WEDNESDAY DINNER

6 ounces pork tenderloin, roasted;
salad with 3 cups romaine lettuce,
1 ounce crumbled blue cheese,
¼ cup chopped tomatoes,
and 2 teaspoons Caesar dressing   8nc

SNACKS

String cheese with 5 black olives   1 nc
1 medium dill pickle   2 nc

***

THURSDAY BREAKFAST

2 slices bacon;
2 eggs, scrambled, topped with 2 tablespoons cheese and 2 tablespoons salsa; hot green tea   4 nc

THURSDAY LUNCH

6 ounce chicken breast;
2 tablespoons nut-free pesto sauce;
1 cup hearts of romaine with 1 tablespoon vinaigrette;

iced tea 3 nc

THURSDAY DINNER

6 ounces Shrimp Scampi 1;
salad with 2 cups romaine lettuce and 5 sliced black olives, 2 teaspoons ranch dressing;
iced tea 7 nc

SNACKS

½ cucumber, sliced with 1 tablespoon cream cheese 3.5 nc
1 cup chicken broth 1 nc

***

FRIDAY BREAKFAST

2-egg omelette with spinach and cheddar cheese;
3 slices Canadian bacon;
coffee 5 nc

FRIDAY LUNCH

6 ounces crab salad in ½ avocado;
8 asparagus spears;
diet lemonade 7 nc

FRIDAY DINNER

6 ounce chicken breast;
½ eggplant, broiled with olive oil;
1 cup mixed greens with vinaigrette. 5 nc

SNACKS

½ sliced tomato
1 ounce whole milk mozzarella cheese   3 nc
celery sticks   1 nc

***

SATURDAY BREAKFAST

broccoli and cheese mini egg omelettes (see recipe);
coffee   2.5 nc

SATURDAY LUNCH

1 six-ounce ground turkey patty and 1 tablespoon salsa;
salad of 2 cups romaine lettuce,
1 ounce crumbled feta cheese, and 2 tablespoons vinaigrette
                                                6 nc

SATURDAY DINNER

1 six-ounce salmon steak, grilled, with lemon juice and melted butter;
2 cups mixed greens with 2 teaspoons bleu cheese dressing
                                                5 nc

SNACKS

shrimp cocktail made from 6 medium shrimp, steamed, with sauce made from combination of sugar-free ketchup and horseradish to taste   3 nc

WEEK TWO SHOPPING LIST

MEATS/SEAFOOD: breakfast sausage, cooked shrimp, flat iron steak, Canadian bacon, ground beef, halibut fillet, cauliflower, sliced ham, roast turkey, turkey sausage links, pork tenderloin, bacon, chicken breast, shrimp, crab meat, ground turkey, salmon steak

PRODUCE: dark greens, parsley, bell pepper, mixed salad greens, zucchini, tomato, cherry tomatoes, mushrooms, arugula, cucumber, lemon, celery, spinach, romaine lettuce, hearts of romaine, garlic, avocado, asparagus, eggplant, broccoli

EGGS AND DAIRY: eggs, Swiss cheese, cheddar cheese, bleu cheese, cream cheese, butter, cream, Monterey jack cheese, sour cream, string cheese, whole milk mozzarella cheese, feta cheese,

OTHER: ranch, bleu cheese, and Caesar dressings, dill pickle spears, green salsa, canned tuna, mayonnaise, sun-dried tomatoes packed in olive oil, black olives, chicken broth, dill pickles, salsa (no added sugar), nut free pesto, sugar-free ketchup, horseradish

Phase Two--Ongoing Weight Loss

SUNDAY BREAKFAST:

2 eggs, poached, topped with 1 small sliced tomato and 2 tablespoons hollandaise sauce;
3 slices Canadian bacon;
hot tea   5.4 nc

SUNDAY LUNCH

Chicken kebab made with 4 ounces cubed chicken,
½ cubed green pepper,
3 mushrooms,
and ⅓ cubed red onion;
2 cups mixed greens with vinaigrette dressing;
2 slices cantaloupe with ½ cup cottage cheese;
mineral water   9.1 nc

SUNDAY DINNER

6 ounce chicken breast stuffed with ½ cup ricotta cheese, wrapped in 1 slice ham;
½ cup spinach and 2 tablespoons pine nuts, sautéd in olive oil

SNACKS

1 ounce almonds	3.6 nc
celery stalk wrapped in 2 slices of prosciutto	1 nc

***

MONDAY BREAKFAST

2 slices bacon topped with sautéed mushrooms,
two slices tomato, and ⅛ cup grated Monterey Jack cheese;
coffee   4.2 nc

MONDAY LUNCH

Asian roll-ups with chicken and peanut sauce (see recipe);
jasmine tea   8 nc

MONDAY DINNER

2 four-oz lamb chops; 8 asparagus spears, grilled and brushed with melted butter;
2 cups mixed greens with 1 ounce crumbled bleu cheese and lite balsamic vinaigrette dressing;
sparkling water   9 nc

SNACKS

1 hard boiled egg	1 nc
½ cup cottage cheese with ½ cup raspberries	3 nc

***

TUESDAY BREAKFAST

Breakfast stuffed pepper, Mexican-style (see recipe);
coffee   5.1 nc

TUESDAY LUNCH

6 ounces cold roast chicken, broccoli and arugula salad (see recipe);   8.9 nc

TUESDAY DINNER

Roast beef au jus;
1/2 cup cauliflower with cheese sauce;
2 cups mixed greens with 1/2 sliced cucumber;
1 ounce chopped hazelnuts, vinaigrette;
iced tea   8.5 nc

SNACKS

avocado salsa (see recipe)   3.6 nc
½ cup cottage cheese with ½ cup raspberries 6 nc

***

WEDNESDAY BREAKFAST

2 eggs baked in ham cups (2 slices) ;
two slices honeydew melon;
coffee   4.9 nc

WEDNESDAY LUNCH

homemade chicken vegetable soup;
¼ cup sliced strawberries;
sparkling water   10.7 nc

WEDNESDAY DINNER

1 six-ounce salmon fillet, grilled;
½ cup snow peas sautéed with ½ cup bok choy and drizzled with sesame oil;
2 cups mixed greens with 2 teaspoons ranch dressing; iced tea with lemon   7.5 nc

SNACKS

2 tablespoons mixed nuts   3 nc
½ cup Greek yogurt with ¼ cup raspberries   5 nc

***

THURSDAY BREAKFAST

Two poached eggs with two slices Canadian bacon;
½ cup Greek yogurt with ¼ cup blueberries. 9 nc

THURSDAY LUNCH

Salad with spinach, bleu cheese crumbles, pistachios, and bacon; bacon vinaigrette;
diet soda   4.2 nc

THURSDAY DINNER

6 ounce grilled top sirloin beef steak;
2 cups mixed green salad with bleu cheese dressing;
2 slices grilled eggplant;
½ cup sautéed mushrooms and onions;
iced tea   10.4 nc

SNACKS

¼ cup strawberries   2.7 nc
2 tablespoons macadamia nuts   2.3 nc

***

FRIDAY BREAKFAST

½ cup Greek yogurt with 2 tablespoons sliced almonds and ¼ cup blueberries;
2 hard boiled eggs;
coffee

FRIDAY LUNCH

6 ounces grilled chicken breast seasoned with chili powder and cumin sliced over 2 cups mixed greens;
½ small tomato, chopped;
1 ounce pepper jack cheese, grated; ranch dressing;
ice water   6.5 nc

FRIDAY DINNER

6 ounces baked flounder; ½ cup sliced red bell pepper;
½ cup snow peas;
1 cup stir-fried bok choy and 1 tablespoon sesame seeds;
2 cups mixed greens;
½ cup beans sprouts; ginger dressing;
iced tea   14 nc

SNACKS

¼ cup cottage cheese and 1 tablespoon walnuts   6.5 nc
¼ cup strawberries with 2 tablespoons whipped cream 3.7 nc

***

SATURDAY BREAKFAST

2 egg omelette with ¼ cup grated cheese and ½ sliced avocado;
½ grilled tomato;
coffee   11.4 nc

SATURDAY LUNCH

2 slices (each) salami, ham, and provolone cheese with mustard, wrapped in a Romaine lettuce leaf;
¼ cup honeydew cubes;
diet soda   6.5 nc

SATURDAY DINNER.

1 six-ounce grilled ham steak;
½ cup mashed turnips;
1 cup mixed greens with vinaigrette;

½ cup raspberries, sliced, with whipped cream   11 nc

SNACKS

1 hard boiled egg   1 nc
½ cup cottage cheese with ½ cup raspberries   3 nc

WEEK ONE SHOPPING LIST

MEATS/SEAFOOD: Canadian bacon, chicken breasts, sliced ham, prosciutto, chicken breast tenderloins, bacon, lamb chops, pork and beef chorizo, 80 percent lean ground beef, roast chicken, beef roast, sliced ham, salmon filet

PRODUCE: tomatoes, lemons, green bell pepper, white mushrooms, red onion, mixed salad greens, cantaloupe, spinach, celery, ginger, avocado, cucumber, jicama, cilantro, asparagus, raspberries, red bell pepper, hazelnuts, pear, broccoli slaw mix, baby arugula, carrot, cauliflower, honeydew melon, green beans, strawberries, snow peas, bok choy, pistachios

EGGS AND DAIRY: eggs, cottage cheese, ricotta cheese, Monterey Jack cheese, butter, bleu cheese, Swiss cheese

OTHER: olive oil, pine nuts, almonds, tamari, rice vinegar, liquid stevia, sushi nori, creamy peanut butter, sriracha sauce, canola oil, light balsamic vinegar, sugar-free maple syrup, Dijon mustard, apple cider vinegar (or sherry vinegar), sesame oil, ranch dressing

WEEK TWO

SUNDAY BREAKFAST:

Two poached eggs with one cup sautéed spinach and hollandaise sauce; two sausage patties;
coffee   4 nc

SUNDAY LUNCH

4 slices of roast beef wrapped around 2 ounces crumbled bleu cheese and 1 cup watercress; roasted zucchini chips; mineral water   8 nc

SUNDAY DINNER

6 ounces Italian sausage sautéed with ½ cup sliced green bell pepper and ½ cup sliced red onion;
2 cups Romaine lettuce with Caesar dressing;
½ cup raspberries; iced tea   13 nc

SNACKS

1 ounce macadamia nuts   1 nc

***

MONDAY BREAKFAST

Blackberry smoothie (see recipe)   6.5 nc

MONDAY LUNCH

Salmon fillet; 1 cup baby spinach leaves with 1 tablespoon crushed walnuts,
2 tablespoons crumbled feta cheese and 5 green olives, drizzled with oil;
diet soda   3.1 nc

MONDAY DINNER

6 ounce sirloin steak;
1 cup broccoli florets steamed with 2 ounces melted cheddar cheese;
2 cups mixed greens with bleu cheese dressing;
iced tea   8 nc

SNACKS

½ cup jicama with 1 tablespoon
lite balsamic vinaigrette   6.7 nc
Swiss cheese cheese and ham rollups;   2.4 nc

***

TUESDAY BREAKFAST

2- egg omelette with chopped breakfast sausage and goat cheese;
¼ cup blueberries;
coffee   7 nc

TUESDAY LUNCH

6 ounces smoked salmon with ½ sliced avocado and 1 tablespoon cream cheese;
1 cup mixed greens with ¼ cup chopped celery, vinaigrette dressing;
club soda   10 nc

TUESDAY DINNER

6 ounce turkey patty with 1 tablespoon sugar-free ketchup, 2 ounces shredded cheddar cheese and one cup arugula; ½ cup baked spaghetti squash;
1 cup mixed greens;
½ cup chopped radishes, and 2 teaspoons ranch dressing;
iced tea   9.5 nc

SNACKS

handful of almonds   3.6 nc

***

WEDNESDAY BREAKFAST

zucchini frittata;
2 slices cantaloupe;
coffee   7.3 nc

WEDNESDAY LUNCH

minestrone soup;
5 buffalo chicken wings;
club soda   13 nc

WEDNESDAY DINNER

6 ounces baked halibut;
1 cup Greek salad with dressing;

½ cup green beans;
iced tea   6.4 nc
SNACKS

1 ounce cream cheese with ½ celery stalk   1.6 nc

***

THURSDAY BREAKFAST

Omelette with spinach and cream cheese;
coffee   4 nc

THURSDAY LUNCH

5 ounces canned tuna, mixed with 1 tablespoon mayonnaise, chopped celery, olives, and cherry tomatoes;
ice water   10 nc

THURSDAY DINNER

Beef and asparagus stir fry; broccoli, daikon, and pepper salad; Swiss chard sautéed with bacon;
iced tea   16.5 nc

SNACK

1 ounce hard cheese   1 nc

***

FRIDAY BREAKFAST

Smoked salmon frittata with asparagus;
coffee   18 nc

FRIDAY LUNCH

Chicken and pistachios on 2 cups mixed greens with light balsamic vinaigrette;
club soda   6 nc

FRIDAY DINNER

6 ounces grilled tuna steak; roasted eggplant and peppers salad;
iced tea   6 nc

SNACKS

½ avocado   2 nc

***

SATURDAY BREAKFAST

2 poached eggs over broiled half tomato;
coffee   4 nc

SATURDAY LUNCH

Turkey roll ups with Boston lettuce and dill pickle spears; mixed greens with dressing;
diet soda   7 nc

SATURDAY DINNER

6 ounce grilled tuna steak with stir-fried bok choy,

1/2 cup bean sprouts,
¼ cup water chestnuts and 1 tablespoon soy sauce, sprinkled with sesame seeds;
¼ cup raspberries and ½ cup Greek yogurt   12 nc

SNACKS

2 ounces macadamia nuts	2.3 nc
hummus with raw vegetables	7 nc

WEEK TWO SHOPPING LIST

MEATS/SEAFOOD: breakfast sausage, sliced roast beef, Italian sausage, salmon fillet, tuna steak, ham slices, smoked salmon, ground turkey, halibut, beef for stir fry, bacon, chicken breast, roast turkey slices, sirloin steak

PRODUCE: spinach, watercress, pistachios, bell pepper, red onion, Romaine lettuce, raspberries, blueberries, blackberries, baby spinach, walnuts, macadamia nuts, bok choy, bean sprouts, sesame seeds, jicama, avocado, mixed salad greens, celery, arugula, spaghetti squash, radishes, carrots, zucchini, cantaloupe, green beans, cherry tomatoes, mozzarella cheese, raspberries, asparagus, broccoli, daikon radish, Swiss chard, red bell pepper, pistachios, eggplant, portabella mushroom, tomatoes,

EGGS AND DAIRY: eggs, butter, bleu cheese, cottage cheese, feta cheese, Greek yogurt, Swiss cheese slices, goat cheese, cream cheese, cheddar cheese, parmesan cheese

OTHER: Caesar dressing, green olives, water chestnuts, soy sauce, light balsamic vinegar, olive oil, ranch dressing, canned tuna, mayonnaise, black olives, hummus, dill pickle spears, bleu cheese dressing

Phases 3 and 4

SUNDAY BREAKFAST:

Cowboy breakfast skillet (see recipe);
coffee   12 nc

SUNDAY LUNCH

Bacon, lettuce, and tomato sandwich with 3 slices bacon, mayo, and low carb multigrain bread;
diet soda   8.5 nc

SUNDAY DINNER
8 ounces halibut topped with ½ cup sautéed scallions;
2 cups mixed greens;
½ cup endive and vinaigrette; \
1 cup sugar-free fruit-flavored gelatin with
whipped cream   6.6 nc

SNACKS

2 tablespoons almonds and
2 ounces brie cheese   3.7 nc
1 cup tomato juice   8 nc

***

MONDAY BREAKFAST

6 ounce steak and 2 eggs, any style;
1 tangerine;
coffee   8.8 nc

MONDAY LUNCH

Portobello mushroom stuffed with spinach and Parmesan cheese;
½ tomato, sliced;
iced tea   7 nc

MONDAY DINNER

1 six-ounce snapper fillet; eight steamed asparagus spears with butter;
2 cups mixed greens,
1 ounce shaved parmesan cheese, and Caesar dressing;
iced tea   6 nc

SNACK

Chocolate "pudding" made with ¼ cup pureed ricotta cheese,
1 tablespoon unsweetened cocoa powder,
and Splenda to taste   11 nc

***

TUESDAY BREAKFAST

1 slice toast from low-carb multigrain bread,
cream cheese;
2 slices honeydew melon   9 nc

TUESDAY LUNCH

1 cup tomato juice, roast beef salad with Swiss cheese, celery, and bleu cheese dressing;   14 nc

TUESDAY DINNER

6 ounces chicken parmigiana;
2 cups salad with chopped olives, radishes, and Italian dressing
   13 nc

SNACKS

Deviled egg   .5 nc

***

WEDNESDAY BREAKFAST

¼ cup blueberries with 2 ounces mascarpone cheese and 2 tablespoons chopped walnuts;
1 hard boiled egg;
herbal tea   7.5 nc

WEDNESDAY LUNCH

6 ounces grilled chicken; lentil salad with green pepper, onion, celery, and vinaigrette   11 nc

WEDNESDAY DINNER

Braised short ribs with horseradish sauce;

½ cup roasted brussels sprouts;
1 cup mixed greens with choice of dressing;
iced tea   17 nc

SNACKS

½ cup cottage cheese with ¼ cup blueberries   8 nc

***

THURSDAY BREAKFAST

2 scrambled eggs with 2 ounces grated cheddar cheese topped with 1 tablespoon salsa;
¼ cup cherries;
coffee   7.8 nc

THURSDAY LUNCH

1 cup vegetable broth; chicken salad in tomato;
zucchini- parmesan chips;
diet soda   12.7 nc

THURSDAY DINNER

6 ounces scallops wrapped in bacon and grilled on skewers;
artichokes with lemon butter;
club soda   11.7 nc

SNACK

2 ounces brie cheese with celery sticks   4 nc

FRIDAY BREAKFAST

Frittata made with eggs, sausage, zucchini, fontina cheese, and sausage;
½ broiled tomato;
coffee   7.1 nc

FRIDAY LUNCH

6 ounce ground turkey patty with 2 ounces Swiss cheese; acorn squash with spiced applesauce and maple drizzle (see recipe);
ice water   12 nc

FRIDAY DINNER

6 ounces pot roast;
½ cup sautéed yellow squash;
2 cups arugula with chopped green beans and vinaigrette dressing;
iced tea   9 nc

SNACK

½ apple with 1 tablespoon peanut butter   13.5 nc

***

SATURDAY BREAKFAST

½ cup fresh pineapple chunks;
2 scrambled eggs;

2 slices Canadian bacon;
coffee   10.7 nc

SATURDAY LUNCH

1 six-ounce chopped sirloin patty topped with 2 tablespoons grated Monterey jack cheese,
½ cup grilled onions, and 2 green chili strips;
¼ cup Mexican slaw;
¼ cup black beans;
diet soda   14 nc

SATURDAY DINNER

1 six-ounce grilled chicken breast;
6 spears asparagus;
½ tomato, sliced;
seltzer   4.9 nc

SNACKS

2 tablespoons hummus with red bell pepper strips 8.4 nc

WEEK ONE SHOPPING LIST

MEAT/SEAFOOD: breakfast sausage, bacon, halibut, 6 ounce steak, 6 ounce red snapper fillet, roast beef slices, chicken breast, 3 pounds short ribs

PRODUCE: sweet potatoes, avocado, cilantro, bibb lettuce, tomato, scallions, mixed salad greens, endive, almonds, brie cheese, portobello mushroom, spinach, tangerine, asparagus, honeydew melon, celery, radishes, blueberries, walnuts, lentils, green bell pepper, onion, brussels sprouts, fennel, carrot, garlic, scallions, 4 artichokes, 4 lemons, acorn squash

EGGS AND DAIRY: eggs, butter, Monterey Jack cheese, heavy whipping cream, Parmesan cheese, ricotta cheese, cream cheese, Swiss cheese, mozzarella cheese, low-carb marinara sauce, mascarpone cheese, cottage cheese,

OTHER: hot sauce, low-carb multigrain bread, mayonnaise, sugar-free fruit flavored gelatin, tomato juice, Caesar dressing, bleu cheese dressing, unsweetened cocoa powder, Splenda, olives, low-carb Italian dressing, dry red wine, 14 ounce can beef broth, allspice, whole wheat flour, sour cream, prepared white horseradish, coriander seed, unsweetened applesauce; ground cinnamon, sugar-free maple syrup

WEEK TWO

SUNDAY BREAKFAST:

2 egg omelette with spinach and feta cheese;
2 halves small tomato, broiled;
1 cup tomato juice   11 nc

SUNDAY LUNCH

Ham, Swiss cheese, and asparagus rollups;
1 cup chicken consommé with sliced mushrooms;
ice water   8 nc

SUNDAY DINNER

6 ounces grilled salmon with lemon butter;
½ cup roasted green beans;
2 cups mixed greens with dressing of choice;
iced tea   7.5 nc

SNACK

Carrot sticks with 2 tablespoons cream cheese   8.1 nc

***

MONDAY BREAKFAST

Zucchini frittata,
2 slices cantaloupe,
coffee   8 nc

MONDAY LUNCH

6 ounce ground turkey patty;
½ cup coleslaw;
1 medium plum;
diet soda   15.2 nc

MONDAY DINNER

Grilled 6 ounce tuna steak;
2 cups baby spinach, cucumber, and tomato salad with choice of dressing;
⅓ cup roasted cauliflower;
club soda   10.4 nc

SNACKS

½ apple   10 nc

***

TUESDAY BREAKFAST

Smoked salmon and cream cheese with onions, tomatoes, and capers;
1 slice low carb multigrain toast with butter;
coffee   9 nc

TUESDAY LUNCH

Turkey, Swiss cheese, and dill pickle spears rolled in bibb lettuce leaves;
¼ cup carrot salad;
½ cup sliced strawberries;
iced water   11.5 nc

TUESDAY DINNER

Roast pork; 1 cup mixed greens, chopped bell peppers, cucumber, and tomatoes with dressing;
½ cup sautéed zucchini and onions;
club soda   9 nc

SNACK

2 ounces walnuts   2 nc

***

WEDNESDAY BREAKFAST

½ cup ricotta cheese with ½ cup sliced strawberries;
1 slice buttered low carb multigrain toast;

coffee   11 nc

WEDNESDAY LUNCH

Tomato stuffed with ½ cup chicken salad;
¼ cup red seedless grapes;
iced tea   14.1 nc

WEDNESDAY DINNER

6 ounces halibut fillet; stir fry with onions, edamame, zucchini, and bell peppers;
2 slices honeydew,   11 nc

SNACKS

1 ounce macadamia nuts   2.3 nc

***

THURSDAY BREAKFAST

2 eggs, any style, with 2 slices Canadian bacon;
1 apricot;
coffee   5.4 nc

THURSDAY LUNCH

1 cup chicken consommé, tomato stuffed with shrimp salad, 2 cups mixed green salad and dressing;
diet soda   9 nc

THURSDAY DINNER

Grilled steak with roasted portobello mushroom;
1 cup okra, grilled on skewer;
iced water   11.4nc

SNACKS

2 tablespoons hummus with celery sticks   5.5 nc

***

FRIDAY BREAKFAST

2 poached eggs, 2 turkey sausage patties,
1 ounce pepper jack cheese;
¼ cup mango chunks;
coffee   9 nc

FRIDAY LUNCH

4 ounces smoked turkey slices and Swiss cheese in sandwich of low carb multigrain bread with mustard, dill pickle slices, and lettuce; one half of apple;
iced water   18 nc

FRIDAY DINNER

Green bell pepper stuffed with 6 ounces ground beef browned with chopped onion and cremini mushrooms;
½ cup cottage cheese;
diet soda   16.5 nc

SNACKS

2 tablespoons almonds   3.6 nc

***

SATURDAY BREAKFAST

2 poached eggs, 1 ounce Swiss cheese, 1 or 2 slices tomato on bed of ½ cup cooked kale with 2 tablespoons hollandaise sauce;
1 tangerine;
coffee   13.3 nc

SATURDAY LUNCH

Crab salad in ½ avocado;
½ cup steamed carrots;
iced water   12.5 nc

SATURDAY DINNER

1 six-ounce pork chop with ½ cup unsweetened applesauce;
½ cup coleslaw;
iced tea   20 nc

SNACK

½ cucumber with 2 tablespoons cream cheese   2.5 nc

WEEK TWO SHOPPING LIST

    MEATS/SEAFOOD: ham slices, salmon fillet, ground turkey, tuna steak, smoked salmon, roast turkey slices, pork roast, chicken breast, halibut fillet, Canadian bacon, shrimp, beef steak, turkey sausage, sliced smoked turkey, ground beef, pork chop, crab salad,

PRODUCE: tomato, baby spinach, asparagus, white mushrooms, lemon, green beans, mixed salad greens, carrots, zucchini, cantaloupe, cabbage, plums, cucumber, cauliflower, apple, strawberries, bibb lettuce, green bell peppers, walnuts, red seedless grapes, edamame, honeydew melon, macadamia nuts, apricot, portobello mushroom, okra, celery, mango, onion, cremini mushrooms, almonds, kale, tangerine, lemon

EGGS AND DAIRY: eggs, butter, feta cheese, Swiss cheese, cream cheese, ricotta cheese, pepper jack cheese, cottage cheese

OTHER: tomato juice, chicken consommé, salad dressings, mayonnaise, capers, low-carb multigrain bread, dill pickle spears, hummus, sandwich dill pickles, unsweetened applesauce

RECIPES FOR EACH PHASE

It's not hard at all to find all kinds of recipes that fit in with the Atkins 20 diet and your personal preferences. Of course, there are plenty of cookbooks dedicated to Atkins and low carb recipes, but you'll also find recipes on plenty of food websites, including Pinterest. The recipes here are designed to give you just a taste of how to cook Atkins-style. This should be a good jumping off place for you to design your own plan.

Phase 1 Recipes

Egg and Sausage Nibbles

Adapted from marksdailyapple.com   Makes 4 large or 6 small squares

Calories: 375 • Fat: 20g • Net carbs: 5.3g • Protein: 25 g

Ingredients

- 1 small bunch of dark greens, such as kale, Swiss chard, beet greens or spinach
- 1-2 cups uncooked sausage, crumbled
- 8-10 eggs
- small bunch parsley

Directions

1. Preheat the oven to 375º F.
2. Slice the greens into thin strips. Sauté in oil or butter over medium heat for several minutes, then add the crumbled sausage.

Continue to sauté until sausage is basically cooked, then turn off heat.
3. Whisk the eggs then stir in the parsley, kale and sausage. Pour into a greased 8×8 pan.
4. Bake 20-25 minutes.
Let cool slightly before cutting into squares.

Broccoli and Cheese Mini Egg Omelettes

Adapted from skinnytaste.com   Makes 4 servings (2 omelettes)

Calories: 167 • Fat: 8.5 g • Net carbs: 2.5 g • Protein: 18 g

Ingredients:

- 4 cups broccoli florets
- 4 whole large eggs
- 1 cup egg whites
- 1/4 cup shredded cheddar
- 1/4 cup grated pecorino Romano cheese
- 1 tsp olive oil
- salt and fresh pepper   to taste
- cooking spray

Directions

1. Preheat oven to 350°.
2. Steam broccoli with a little water for about 6-7 minutes. When broccoli is cooked, chop into smaller pieces and add olive oil, salt and pepper. Mix well.
3. Spray a standard size non-stick muffin tin with cooking spray and spoon broccoli mixture evenly into 9 cups.
4. In a medium bowl, beat egg whites with eggs, and add grated cheese, salt and pepper.

5. Pour into the greased tins over broccoli until a little more than 3/4 full. Top with grated cheddar and bake in the oven until cooked, about 20 minutes. Serve immediately.
6. Any leftovers can be wrapped in plastic wrap and stored in the refrigerator up to 3 days.

Mexican-style Eggs on Canadian Bacon

Adapted from atkins.com　　　　　　　　Makes 4 servings

Calories: 287 • Fat: 20.2g • Net carbs: 2.5 g • Protein: 23 g

Ingredients

- 6 ounces ground beef (80% lean / 20% fat)
- 1/2 cup green chili peppers (canned)
- 1/4 tsp garlic powder
- 1 tsp chili powder
- 1/4 tsp cumin
- 1/4 tsp leaf oregano
- 1/4 tsp salt
- 1/4 tsp black pepper
- 4 slices Canadian bacon
- 4 large eggs (whole)
- 1/2 cup, shredded cheddar cheese
- 4 sprigs cilantro

Directions

1. Spray a medium skillet with non-stick cooking spray and brown the beef over medium heat.

2. Stir in chilis, garlic powder, chili powder, cumin, oregano, salt, and pepper. Cook 5-10 minutes to blend the flavors.
3. Place the slices of Canadian bacon over the top of the beef mixture to warm.
   Remove pan from heat and set aside.
4. In a separate skillet, scramble eggs until set. (If you prefer, you can fry or poach eggs and place on top of the beef mixture in step 5.)
5. Place 1 piece of warmed Canadian bacon on each plate, top with a quarter of the beef mixture and a quarter of the eggs. Sprinkle with cheese and chopped cilantro.

Maple-Dijon Vinaigrette

Adapted from Atkins.com   Makes eight 2 tablespoon servings

Calories: 126 • Fat: 13.5g • Net carbs: .3 g

Ingredients

- 1/2 cup extra virgin olive oil
- 2 oz sugar-free maple flavored syrup
- 4 tablespoons red wine vinegar
- 4 tsps Dijon mustard
- 1 tsp salt (optional)
- 1/2 tsp black pepper (optional)

Directions

Whisk all ingredients together and season with additional salt and freshly ground black pepper to taste. Keeps in the refrigerator for up to two weeks.

Crispy Carnitas

Adapted from marksdailyapple   Makes 6 servings

Calories: 485 • Fat: 36.7g • Net carbs: 1.7 g • Protein: 34.8 g

Ingredients

- 3 to 4 pounds boneless pork shoulder/butt cut into five pieces.
- 1 1/2 teaspoons salt
- 1 teaspoon cumin
- 1 teaspoon chili powder
- 1 cinnamon stick
- 1 bay leaf
- 4 garlic cloves, thinly sliced
- 1 onion, chopped
- Water for braising

Directions

1. Preheat the oven to 350 °F.
2. Mix together the salt, cumin, and chili powder and rub into the meat.
3. Place pork pieces in a single layer in a large Dutch oven and add the onion and the remaining spices. Add enough water to almost cover the meat.
4. Let braise uncovered in oven for 3 to 3 1/2 hours. Stir the meat occasionally as it cooks. The pork is done when it's slightly browned, very tender, and most of the liquid is gone.
5. Remove pork to a cutting board and cut or shred it into thin strips.
6. Recipe can be made ahead up to this point. Refrigerate until almost time to serve.
7. Remove the cinnamon stick and bay leaf, and return the shredded to the pot, or spread out on a baking sheet with any leftover liquid. Place it back in the oven and roast,

tossing occasionally, until the meat becomes dark and crispy.

The carnitas can also be cooked on the stovetop or in a slow cooker with about ½ cup of water. Cook the meat until tender and then transfer to the oven to brown.

Creamy Soup with Mini Turkey Meatballs

Adapted from Sparkrecipes   Makes 2 servings

Calories: 382 • Fat: 27.8g • Net carbs: 3g • Protein: 27.2g

Ingredients

- 1 tbsp. unsalted butter
- 1 minced clove garlic
- 1 ¼ oz chopped broccoli
- about 4 medium white mushrooms, chopped
- 8 oz. lean ground turkey
- 1 extra large egg
- 1 tablespoon chicken bouillon
- ¼ cup heavy cream
- spices to taste for meatballs (suggestion: chili powder, oregano, ground ginger, ground curry, turmeric, basil)
- enough water to cook mini-meatballs in.

Directions

1. Bring water to a boil.
2. In a small bowl, combine ground turkey, egg, and spices. Working with tablespoon-sized scoops, form the mixture into small balls and set aside.
3. Melt butter in medium saucepan and add garlic. Stir over medium heat for about 30 seconds, then add the mushrooms. Allow them to cook down and add the chopped broccoli.

4. Add about 5 cups boiling water to the sautéed veggies. Bring to boil again and add the bouillon. Water can be increased or decreased according to taste.
5. Drop the meatballs into the boiling soup mixture. Let cook for about 10 minutes, then add the heavy cream. Taste and adjust seasoning, if necessary.

Shrimp Fried "Rice"

Adapted from *Cooking Light* magazine Makes four 1-cup servings

Calories: 269• Fat: 17g • Net carbs: 6g • Protein: 20g

Ingredients:

- 3 tablespoons toasted sesame oil, divided
- 10 oz. medium shrimp, peeled and deveined
- 5 large eggs, lightly beaten
- 1 cup sliced green onions, divided
- 16 oz. fresh or frozen riced cauliflower
- ½ t freshly ground black pepper
- ¼ t kosher salt

Directions

1. Heat 1 ½ teaspoons sesame oil in a large nonstick skillet over medium high. Add shrimp ; cook 3 minutes. Remove shrimp from pan.
2. Return pan to medium high. Add 1 ½ teaspoons oil. Add eggs,; cook 2 minutes or until almost set, stirring once. Fold cooked eggs in half; remove from pan. Cool and cut into ½ inch pieces.
3. Heat remaining 2 tablespoons of oil in pan over medium-high. Add ¾ cup of green onion, cauliflower, cook 5 minutes without stirring, or until browned. Stir in shrimp,

eggs, salt, and pepper. Top with remaining ¼ cup green onions.

Faux Mashed "Potatoes"

Makes 1 serving

Calories: 80 • Fat: 5.5g • Net carbs: 4g • Protein: 2.4g

Ingredients

- 1 cup cauliflower florets
- 1 tablespoon butter
- 2 tablespoons heavy cream
- sea salt
- ground pepper

Directions

1. Steam cauliflower florets until tender.
2. Puree with butter and cream.
3. Season to taste with salt and pepper.

Avocado Salsa

Adapted from atkins.com   Makes 4 servings

Calories: 86.4• Fat: 6.7g • Net carbs: 3.6g • Protein: 1.3g

Ingredients

- 1 small tomato, chopped
- ⅛ cup cilantro, chopped
- 1 small red onion, diced
- ½ jalapeño pepper, seeded and minced (wear rubber gloves to avoid burning skin, and do not touch face or eyes)
- 1 avocado, peeled and chopped
- 2 tablespoons fresh lime juice

- ⅛ teaspoon salt
- ⅛ teaspoon black pepper

Directions

1. Place avocado in a serving bowl. Add the onion, jalapeño and lime juice to the avocado and gently combine; do not mash.
2. Fold in chopped tomato and cilantro and season with salt and pepper.
3. Cover and refrigerate until ready to serve.

Chorizo With Lemon-Mayo Dip

Adapted from atkins.com   Makes 4 servings
Calories: 805.3 • Fat: 77.9g • Net carbs: 2.8g • Protein: 21.9g

Ingredients

- 6 four-inch links pork and beef chorizo
- 1 tablespoon extra-virgin olive oil
- 1 cup mayonnaise
- 2 tablespoons lemon juice
- 1 tablespoon lemon peel
- ½ clove garlic, minced
- 2 medium stalks celery, cut into sticks

Directions

1. Slice chorizo into 1/2-inch rounds.
2. Heat oil in a large skillet over medium heat. Cook chorizo 5 to 7 minutes, turning once, until browned on both sides. Remove from pan and drain on paper towels.
3. Place mayonnaise, lemon juice, zest and garlic in a mixing bowl. Stir well to combine. Serve chorizo with celery sticks and mayonnaise.

PHASE 2 RECIPES

Baked Eggs and Asparagus
Adapted from Atkins.com   Makes 1 serving

Calories: 473 • Fat: 40g • Net carbs: 3.6g • Protein: 21g

Ingredients

- 8 smallish asparagus spears
- ¼ cup heavy cream
- 2 large eggs
- 2 tablespoons almond meal flour
- 1 tablespoon grated Parmesan cheese
- ⅛ teaspoon minced garlic
- ⅛ tsp Black Pepper

Directions

1. Preheat oven to 400°F. Prepare a small spread a small amount of oil in a ramekin and set aside.
2. Steam the asparagus spears for 2 minutes until tender-crisp. Drain and run under cold water. Pat dry and arrange in the prepared ramekin.
3. Drizzle cream over the asparagus and crack the eggs over all.
4. In a small bowl blend together the almond meal, Parmesan cheese, garlic, and black pepper. Sprinkle over the eggs and place in oven.
5. Cook for 5-10 minutes, depending upon how firm you like your eggs. The cream will puff over the edges of the eggs and the topping should be golden brown.

Blackberry smoothie

Adapted from atkins.com   Makes 1 serving

Calories: 210 • Fat: 6.9g • Net carbs: 6 • Protein: 25g

Ingredients

- ¼ cup frozen blackberries
- 1 cup unsweetened coconut, almond, or soy milk
- 1 oz vanilla whey protein
- 1 tablespoon ground golden flaxseed meal
- ¼ tsp cinnamon
- pinch ground allspice
- ½ teaspoon vanilla extract

Directions

Combine the frozen blackberries, milk, protein powder, flax meal, vanilla, and spices in a blender. Blend until smooth.

Breakfast Stuffed Pepper, Mexican Style

Adapted from atkins.com   Makes 1 serving

Calories: 326 • Fat: 24g • Net carbs: 5g • Protein: 21g

Ingredients

- 1 oz pork and beef chorizo
- 1 ounce 80% lean ground beef
- 2 tablespoons chopped onion
- ¼ oz cheddar cheese, grated
- 1 large egg, beaten
- 1 medium sweet red peppers, cut in half lengthwise, seeds and white ribs removed

Directions

1. Preheat oven to 400°F and line a baking sheet with foil.

2. In a pan over medium heat, cook chorizo and ground beef, crumbling meat while it cooks. Drain off excess fat.
3. Place cooked meat mixture in mixing bowl and combine with the onion, cheese and egg.
4. Fill pepper half with the meat mixture and place on the prepared baking sheet. Bake for 25-30 minutes and serve hot.

Arugula, Pear and Hazelnut Salad

Adapted from Atkins.com   Makes 4 servings

Calories: 252 • Fat: 21g • Net carbs: 8g • Protein: 8g

Ingredients

- 10 oz arugula
- ½ cup gorgonzola cheese, crumbled
- 1 medium pear
- 40 hazelnuts
- 4 tablespoons maple-Dijon vinaigrette (see recipe, phase 1 section)

1. Toast hazelnuts in a dry skillet for about 15 minutes, or toast on a baking sheet in a 350°F oven, stirring 2-3 times for both methods. Allow to cool and gently rub off outer skin. Coarsely chop, and set aside.
2. Toss dressing with the arugula and Gorgonzola cheese and transfer to serving plates.
3. Arrange the pear slices in a fan on top and sprinkle with chopped hazelnuts.

Asian Roll-ups with Chicken and Peanut Sauce

Adapted from Atkins .com   Makes 2 servings

Losing Weight with Atkins Diet Plan: A Beginner's Guide

Calories: 404 • Fat 23g • Net carbs: 8g • Protein: 31g

Ingredients

- 2 chicken breast tenderloins
- 1 ½ tablespoons tamari
- 1 tablespoon rice vinegar
- 1 teaspoon minced ginger, divided
- liquid stevia
- ½ avocado
- ¼ cucumber with peel
- 2 ½ oz. cup jicama
- 8 sprigs cilantro
- 2 sheets sushi nori
- ½ tablespoon canola oil
- 1 ½ tablespoons natural creamy peanut butter
- 4 tablespoons water
- ¾ teaspoon sriracha sauce

Directions

1. Place tamari, rice vinegar, ginger, and stevia in a plastic zip bag and shake to blend well. Add the chicken tenderloins to the marinade and set aside.
2. While the chicken is marinating, prepare the vegetables. Slice the avocado into 8 long wedges. Cut the cucumber and jicama into sticks measuring about 3 x 1/8 inches.
3. Divide ingredients into 4 equal portions. Set all aside on a cutting board, along with the sprigs of cilantro.
4. Gently fold the nori sheets in half and then tear them in two; set all 4 sheets aside.
5. Place the vegetable oil in a nonstick skillet over medium-high heat. Add the chicken, discarding the remaining marinade. Cook chicken until no longer pink in the center; about 3 minutes per side.

6. Place on the cutting board with the other ingredients and slice each tenderloin into 3 pieces (if you only had 3 tenderloins, cut into an amount that is easily divided by 4). Place a small dish of water next to the assembly line. Set aside.
7. In a small bowl combine the peanut butter, water, 1 ½ teaspoon tamari, remaining ½ teaspoon minced ginger, 3-4 drops stevia and ¾ teaspoon sriracha. Blend until all ingredients are incorporated, adjust seasonings to taste by adding more tamari, ginger, stevia or sriracha.
8. Assembly: Place 1/2 sheet of nori on a flat surface. Place the sliced avocado, cucumber, jicama, and cilantro at a slight angle so they align with the corner of one end of the nori sheet with about 1/2-inch of the corner of the nori sheet sticking out. Dredge the chicken in the peanut sauce and place it on top of the vegetables. Roll, starting at the side where you placed the ingredients, then change direction slightly so that it creates a cone shape, with one end tightly rolled and the other end open. Dip your fingertips in the water bowl, and spread water on the nori sheet at the end corner of the wrap, hold it down a few seconds to seal the wrap in place. Repeat for remaining wraps.
9. Use any remaining sauce for dipping.

PHASE 3 AND 4 RECIPES

COWBOY BREAKFAST SKILLET

Adapted from health-bent.com   Makes 5 servings

Calories: 355 • Fat: 17g • Net carbs: 12g • Protein: 22g

Ingredients

- 1 lb breakfast sausage
- 2 medium sweet potatoes, diced
- eggs
- 1 avocado, peeled and cubed
- handful cilantro, chopped
- hot sauce
- ½ cup grated cheese (optional)
- salt and pepper to taste

Directions

1. Preheat oven to 400°F.
2. In a cast iron or other oven-safe skillet, crumble and brown the sausage over medium heat. Use a slotted spoon to remove the sausage and drain on paper towels. Leave as much of the sausage drippings as possible in the skillet.
3. Add the sweet potatoes to the skillet and toss in the sausage grease until cooked through and crispy.
4. Return the sausage to the pan, and with a large spoon, make a depression in the mixture, a "nest" for each egg. Crack your eggs into the nests.
5. Place the skillet into the preheated oven and bake just long enough for the eggs to set, about 5 minutes.
6. Now, turn the oven to broil the top of the eggs for a few minutes, but don't let the yolk cook all the way through– unless you prefer a well-cooked yolk. Remove the pan from the oven and top with avocado, cilantro, and hot sauce.
7. Use a large spoon to scoop out each egg, along with its nest.

Artichokes with Lemon-Butter

Adapted from Atkins.com   Makes 4 servings

Calories: 288• Fat: 23.8g • Net carbs: 10.7g • Protein: 5.4g

Ingredients

- 4 medium artichokes, stems and points trimmed
- 4 lemons
- 2 tablespoons coriander seed
- 2 tablespoons salt
- ½ cup unsalted butter

Directions

1. Bring 4 quarts of water to a boil in a large pot.
2. Cut 3 lemons in half and squeeze juice into water. Add lemon halves, coriander seeds and salt. Place artichokes in the cooking liquid. If necessary, cover them with a heavy plate to keep them from floating. Boil 15 minutes, until a paring knife can be easily inserted at the joint of the stem. Remove artichokes from pot and drain excess water.
3. Melt butter, mix in juice of remaining lemon, salt and pepper.
4. Serve each person one whole artichoke and use butter sauce for dipping.

Braised Short Ribs with Horseradish Sauce

Adapted from *Atkins for Life*   Makes 4 servings

Calories: 402 • Fat: 24g • Net carbs: 7g • Protein: 30.5g

Ingredients

- 3 pounds short ribs
- ½ teaspoon sea salt
- ¼ teaspoon black pepper
- 1 ½ teaspoons canola oil

- 1 cup chopped fennel
- 1 medium carrot, finely diced
- 2 large garlic cloves, minced
- ½ cup plus 2 tablespoons dry red wine
- 1 14 oz can beef broth
- ¼ teaspoon ground allspice
- 2 tablespoons whole wheat flour

For horseradish cream:
- ½ cup sour cream
- 1 tablespoon prepared white horseradish, well drained
- 1 tablespoon thinly sliced scallions

Directions:

1. Preheat oven to 325° F. Sprinkle short ribs with salt and pepper. On the stove, set burner to medium high heat and set Dutch oven on burner. Place half of ribs in Dutch oven and brown well, about 3 to 4 minutes per side. Transfer to a plate and repeat with remaining ribs, removing them when they're browned.
2. Reduce heat to medium. Add oil, fennel, and carrot to Dutch oven and cook for about 3 minutes, or until vegetables are light golden. Add garlic and cook for 1 minute. Add ½ cup wine and simmer for 1 minute. Add ribs to vegetable/wine mixture, stir in broth and allspice. Bring to a boil.
3. Cover and transfer to preheated oven for 2 ¼ to 2 ½ hours, until meat is so tender it falls off the bone.
4. While ribs are braising, prepare horseradish cream. Mix sour cream, horseradish, and scallions. Stir until combined. Store in refrigerator until serving time.
5. When ribs are done, transfer to a bowl. Skim as much fat as possible from the surface of the liquid. (Can be made a

day ahead and refrigerated so that the fat hardens and is easily removed.)
6. Stir remaining 2 tablespoons wine into flour and whisk into cooking liquid. Bring to a boil and simmer 1 to 2 minutes until thickened, stirring frequently. Return ribs to liquid and cook until heated through. Serve with horseradish cream.

Broccoli and Arugula Salad

Adapted from *Cooking Light* magazine   Makes 4 servings
Calories: 120 • Fat: 10 g • Net carbs: 5 g • Protein: 1 g

Ingredients:

- 3 T extra virgin olive oil
- 2 T sherry vinegar or apple cider vinegar
- ½ t black pepper
- ⅜ t kosher salt
- 3 c baby arugula
- 1 ½ c broccoli slaw mix
- 1 c shredded carrot

Directions

1. Combine first 4 ingredients and mix well with a whisk.
2. Mix arugula, broccoli slaw mix, and carrot.
3. Pour dressing over salad and toss lightly until coated.

Acorn Squash with Spiced Applesauce and Maple Drizzle

Adapted from atkins.com

Calories: 73 • Fat: 3.3g • Net carbs: 10g • Protein: .7g

Ingredients

- 1 4 inch acorn squash
- 5 tablespoons unsalted butter
- ½ teaspoon salt
- ½ teaspoon black pepper
- ¾ cup unsweetened applesauce
- ⅛ teaspoon cinnamon
- 1 tablespoon sugar-free maple flavored syrup

Directions

1. Preheat oven to 350°F. Cut squash in half, remove seeds, and then cut into six wedges.
2. Line a sheet pan with aluminum foil. Melt 1 tablespoon butter and brush on squash; sprinkle with salt and pepper, place on pan, and bake in preheated oven until squash is fork tender, about 20 minutes
3. In a small saucepan, heat the applesauce about three minutes. Stir in 2 teaspoons butter and cinnamon, and cook 30 seconds more.
4. Serve squash with a dollop of apple sauce mixture and a drizzle of about 1/2 teaspoon syrup.

A Final Word

From the outset, Dr. Atkins has always made the principles of his low carbohydrate diet very clear in his books, but for some reason, there still seems to be some confusion about what kind of diet it really is. There are still many people out there who believe that Atkins is all about high protein and stuffing yourself with your favorite foods as long as they're on the acceptable foods list. Hopefully, after reading this book, you understand that that is not the case at all. The Atkins approach is a sensible balance of foods that includes a carefully planned restriction of insulin-spiking carbohydrates.

If this is your first experience with the low-carb lifestyle, it's easy to be overwhelmed by all the information that seems to come at you from every direction. It seems like everyone you meet is an expert, and they'll want to give you advice on what they think you're doing wrong. It's okay to listen to them--it's only polite, after all--but in the end, you're the one who knows your body best, so listen to what your body tells you.

If you're a busy person (and who isn't?) you can explore some of the low-carb convenience foods out there. You'll find that Atkins provides many delicious shakes, bars, and meals, and most of them are acceptable from Phase 1 on. Other brands may also be permissible, but you should read the labels carefully to ensure you're buying what you think you are.

Even though it goes without saying, we're going to say it anyway: cutting carbs is not the total answer to good health. Try to avoid carb-free foods that have a lot of chemicals, salts, or other ingredients that can undermine your health. That includes just about all fast food. And don't forget about exercise. Get your body moving and your heart pumping at least 30 minutes a day.

This will be easier as the weight comes off, and you'll probably even begin to enjoy it!

The ball's in your court now. You have the information, the tools, and the motivation. Now is the time to set up the program that will work for you. You're just four phases, or maybe only three, from having the body, the health, and the quality of life that you dream of.

ONE LAST THING... DID YOU ENJOY THE BOOK?

If so, then let me know by leaving a review on Amazon! Reviews are the lifeblood of independent authors. I would appreciate even a few words from you!

If you did not like the book, then please tell me! Email me at lizard.publishing@gmail.com and let me know what you didn't like. Perhaps I can change it. In today's world, a book doesn't have to be stagnant. It should be improved with time and feedback from readers like you. You can impact this book, and I welcome your feedback. Help me make this book better for everyone!

Copyright 2017 by Anna Adams - All rights reserved.

All Rights Reserved. No part of this publication or the information in it may be quoted from or reproduced in any form by means such as printing, scanning, photocopying or otherwise without prior written permission of the copyright holder.

Disclaimer and Terms of Use: Effort has been made to ensure that the information in this book is accurate and complete, however, the author and the publisher do not warrant the accuracy of the information, text and graphics contained within the book due to the rapidly changing nature of science, research, known and unknown facts and internet. The Author and the publisher do not hold any responsibility for errors, omissions or contrary interpretation of the subject matter herein. This book is presented solely for motivational and informational purposes only.

About the Author

Anna Adams has had a life-long love affair with food. Somewhere along the line, she realized that her relationship with food had become toxic, and her health was beginning to suffer. Even so, she was still unwilling to say goodbye to her passion and instead looked for a way to make the relationship work. That's when she discovered Atkins.

Now a firm believer, she has studied all the books and resources on the Atkins diet and in the process she has taken off 20 pounds and is enjoying a much healthier, happier life. She is very grateful, and this book is her way of paying it forward.

Printed in Great Britain
by Amazon